# Don't Diet

# *Live It!*

# Don't Diet —*Live It!*

Successful Weight Control
for Real People
Who Enjoy Real Food

MARY GUAY

WHITE PAPERS PRESS
MARIETTA, GA

# DON'T DIET —*LIVE IT!*

Successful Weight Control for

Real People Who Enjoy Real Food

WHITE PAPERS PRESS

Post Office Box 72294

Marietta, GA 30007-2294

Library of Congress Catalog Card Number 97-97031

**Publisher's Cataloging-in-Publication**
**(Provided by Quality Books, Inc)**

Guay, Mary.
    Don't Diet--live it! : successful weight control for real people who enjoy real food / Mary Guay. -- 1st ed.
    p. cm.
    Includes bibliographical references and index.
    ISBN: 0-9654669-5-7

    1. Weight loss.   I. Title.

RM222.2.G83  1998        613.2'5
                   QB197-41282

Cover design by C. Mayapriya Long, Bookwrights

Printed in the United States of America.

*This book is dedicated to all those who, like me, have struggled with weight loss in a world filled with temptation.*

*This book, as well as many of my endeavors, would not have been possible without twenty years of unqualified support from my husband.*

# Disclaimer

This book is designed to provide information on the subject matter that is addressed. The author and publisher are not engaged in rendering medical advice or other professional services. If medical or other expert assistance is required, you should seek the services of a qualified professional.

It is not the intent of the author or publisher to reprint information in this book that is otherwise available from other sources. You are urged to read and research all issues related to weight control, nutrition and health and use that information for your own individual situation.

This text should be used as a general guide and not as the ultimate source of weight control, nutrition and health. Every effort has been made to make this book as accurate as possible. However, there may be both typographical mistakes and mistakes in content. Also, this book contains information on the subject matter only up to the printing date.

The purpose of this book is to entertain and educate. The author and White Papers Press will have neither liability nor responsibility to any person or entity regarding any loss or damage caused, alleged to be caused, directly or indirectly by the information written in this book.

If you do not wish to be bound by the information above, you may return this book to White Papers Press for a full refund of the purchase price.

# The Author

Mary Guay is a real person who eats real food. She is like you. You will not see her on Oprah, or touring the country in spandex workout gear. She does not (and does not care to) have a personal trainer or personal nutritionist.

Mary is like hundreds of thousands of people who have struggled with weight control in a world filled with temptation. After years of unsuccessful dieting, she fought back. Armed with the latest research in nutrition, and the behavior modification methods shared in this book, she has learned to control her weight without eliminating wonderful foods, and without drugs, fad diets, embarrassing workout sessions, or prepared meals.

Mary earned science degrees in Microbiology and Medical Technology. After working in a medical lab for several years, she is now a writer living in Atlanta with her husband of twenty years, their two teenage sons, two annoying miniature dachshunds, and a perfect cat.

# Contents

# INTRODUCTION

C ongratulations! You may have chosen this book because you are fed up, literally, with your weight and unhealthy lifestyle and are at a low point in your life. But one year from now, you will remember this day as one of the most important and positive days of your life.

I have joked that the ultimate weight control book only needs to contain four words—EAT LESS MOVE MORE. However, we all know this. In order to lose weight, you must consume less calories than you use. Yet, in our

*Throw your heart over the fence and the rest will follow.*
*-Norman Vincent Peale*

complicated society with an abundance of food, weight control is not that simple. If it was, we would all have the bodies we envy. There would not be a multi-billion dollar industry revolving around our obsession to lose weight. Thousands of books, diet aids, supplements, prepackaged meals, drugs, exercise equipment and programs, gyms, videos, surgical procedures and herbs are promoted to help people eat less and move more. Most of us know what it takes to lose weight, but *how we get there and stay there* is the challenge. How to break out of the cycle of overeating and guilt is the key.

That is what this book is about—breaking out of that cycle by moving towards your goal with small, yet certain and achievable lifestyle changes, and transforming a multitude of poor daily eating choices into better choices one by one, bit by bit, and inch by inch. At the same time, your weight will drop ounce by ounce. Most people do not gain their excess weight in a matter of months. More likely, your weight gain was due to many poor eating and lifestyle habits developed over years. Using this same premise, by developing better eating and lifestyle habits over a solid period of time, you can be successful in losing weight and keeping it off. In the same way that your body learned to love high-fat, high-calorie foods, your body will learn to crave nutritious foods. It can be done. With the right skills, you can do it.

The *Live It!* Plan uses the innate human ability to form habits. Habits are powerful behavior regulators. Bad habits can ruin your life, yet good habits can prolong your life. Many poor eating choices are a result of habitual acts rather than a consequence of lack of discipline and will power. Slowly changing these bad habits into healthy habits can bring you results without sacrificing the things you love.

*The* Live It! *Plan breaks the seemingly insurmountable task of weight loss into small, achievable steps.*

The *Live It!* Plan also uses the power of planning. Your current poor lifestyle habits are a result of a lack of planning and control. You certainly did not plan to grow to your current weight. However, it is never too late to take control. Surely you have made many plans in your life—plans for education, for family, vacation and business. There is no reason in the world why you cannot also plan your weight and health. Plans help us anticipate problems and opportunities, and gain control. A plan helps mold your mindset, reinforces your goal, and keeps you on track. Like a business plan, the *Live It!* Plan breaks the seemingly insurmountable task of weight loss into small, achievable steps that cumulatively and deliberately lead to success.

This plan is powerful. There are 52 small changes that all together result in profound lifestyle change. One change per week is discussed and introduced into your lifestyle. The beauty of these changes is that each one is *achievable*. Many of these changes have little to do with eating less or different foods. Some changes will be more challenging for you than others. All result in increased activity, decreased caloric intake and/or a mindset of health. And even though some of these changes are very simple, each time you practice them they reinforce your ultimate goal.

You may think that a year is far too long and you are too impatient to wait that long. How long have you wanted to lose weight? How would you feel if you had started this plan last year? How many quick weight-loss programs have

> *It matters not what goal you seek*
> *Its secret here reposes:*
> *You've got to dig from week to week*
> *To get Results or Roses.*
> *-Edgar Guest*

you endured only to see the pounds return, and sometimes even more than you lost? Quick weight-loss programs rarely result in lifelong weight control. Your body interprets a drastic reduction in calories as a state of starvation. Metabolism slows down. Fat is stored. Your body responds in a very appropriate manner—it reserves energy during the famine. Your body will also stock up on extra reserves when regular eating patterns resume. This results in fatigue, and very quick weight gain when you inevitably abandon the quick weight loss scheme.

No one can remain on a restricted diet forever. At some point you must return to the real world and face those poor eating habits. This is why yo-yo dieters fail. And no one can be expected to change their eating habits overnight. If you started tomorrow on a diet that strictly followed the Food Guide Pyramid, you would feel deprived and hungry. Those cravings would get you. Guilt would creep in, and the old cycle would continue.

A year is not a long time to adjust from a lifetime of poor eating habits to healthy eating habits. One year allows a gradual introduction of these changes and gives your body and attitude time to adjust and accept. Building a better lifestyle is much like building a house—each stage builds on the next, and the care that is invested in each stage directly affects the quality of the final product. A well built house resting on a poorly laid foundation will not stand long. Care and patience with every brick laid results in a house that will last a lifetime.

*Warning: Dates in Calendar are closer than they appear.*
*-Anonymous bumper sticker*

You have decided to make changes. You have taken an active step to control your life, weight and health. You are one step closer to being thinner, healthier and happier. By choosing to *plan* a lifestyle, you have already started on that journey.

The *Live It!* Plan centers on refocusing your lifestyle. This is not a diet. There are no restrictive menus, no pills, no gimmicks. This is a sensible, flexible, achievable, and safe way to gain control of your lifestyle. This is a change in attitude. Take a good look in the mirror. Who you see is responsible for your eating habits now and, more importantly, who you see is the only person who can change those habits. That person is fully deserving of a more healthy, great looking body. This is the only body that you have. And it's a great one. Treat it like gold.

# HOW THE *LIVE IT!* PLAN WORKS

Y ou may worry that you will have to give up a favorite food. This is not necessary. You can eat all the foods that you enjoy. In some cases, you will reduce the quantity of the portions, or reduce the number of times per week in which you eat them, or modify the caloric content. The modifications must be gradual so that your appetite and metabolism will accept the change in lifestyle. Your body will

*Believe it or not, your cravings will change to more nutritious foods.*

have time to adjust to a healthier daily diet. Cravings for high-calorie foods will subside. Believe it or not, your cravings will change to more nutritious foods.

The *Live It!* Plan is modeled on a daily diet based on the latest research in nutrition and the Food Guide Pyramid (discussed in Week 7.) The Food Guide Pyramid recommends a certain number of servings of each category of food. You choose the combination of foods that fit into each category. Diversity is important for a healthy diet—not only the diversity of food, but also the diversity of appetites and dietary needs that we all have. This plan does not prescribe a regimen of daily meals. Your doctor may have provided you with menus, and certainly you have your own favorites. It is important to have diversity in your diet, to maintain nutrition and interest. Foods that may satisfy one person, may be intolerable to another.

Diversity in diet is also important because throughout your life you will be confronted with a variety of foods and situations. You must learn to choose your foods, and modify your behavior in these situations. Diet plans that use packaged meals or supplements do not give you the skills needed to make appropriate choices in the real world. These meals are mainly a lucrative source of income for the distributor. You do not want to be tied to tightly controlled menus and meals. *You* want to be the one in control, not a diet food manufacturer.

*Don't be afraid to give your best to what seemingly are small jobs. Every time you conquer one it makes you that much stronger. If you do the little jobs well, the big ones will tend to take care of themselves.*
*-Dale Carnegie*

This book is meant to be used for an entire year. Each week you will read about one suggested lifestyle change to achieve weight loss and improved health. You will use that entire week to incorporate that change into *your* everyday lifestyle and environment. Many tips are given to ease you into the change. Most changes are easy and painless, yet the cumulative effect of all 52 changes is astounding.

The Appendix contains dozens of suggestions, summarized from the chapters, for food substitutions. Ideally, you should adopt all of these suggestions in your everyday life. I admit that I do not strictly adhere to all of these. Some I practice without exception, some much of the time, and some not at all. We all have different tastes and different lifestyles, so if one is particularly difficult or does not apply to you, you can skip it or adopt a substitution of your own. Just remember that the more you adopt, the quicker you will gain control of your weight. Your goal is to end the year with an arsenal of small changes that together result in a huge impact on your lifestyle.

Each week, focus completely on the task or change for the week. Think of ways that you can incorporate the task into your routine and your environment. As you move forward into the next week, continue to practice the tasks from previous weeks.

*You will end the year with an arsenal of small changes that together result in a huge impact on your lifestyle.*

Skim through the book so that you can envision the coming year. You can read the entire book, but do not try to implement the changes more quickly than suggested. The gradual introduction of these changes is vital to your success. Be deliberate about your commitments and changes, and take your time. Before you know it, the end of the year will be here and you will have either met your goal or you will have the skills and lifestyle that can make that goal a lifelong reality.

Let's get started!

# FIRST QUARTER:

# LAYING A

# FOUNDATION

# WEEK 1: PUT IT IN WRITING

T he first step in modifying your eating habits is to gain a very clear understanding of your present habits. The goal of this first week is to **accurately record everything that you put in your mouth.** Eat as you normally eat. By the end of the week, you should be crystal clear about what goes into your body every day. This act alone will be powerful eye-opener in understanding how those pounds got where they are. The information is vital to establishing a baseline of caloric intake (the amount of calories that you now consume), and to judge your progress. You will refer back to these records months from now and be amazed at what you ate every day. The records can also be an important tool for a healthcare consultation, if you choose to use it this way.

Keeping a food journal is an important first step in taking control of your weight. Here are the keys to make the most of your food journal:

- Find a good recording tool. It is important that you record what you eat in an orderly and convenient way. A sample journal page follows. You can make your own journal, but be sure that it is easy and convenient to use. If you are already using a time planner, you should be able to adapt the pages to include the entries for a food journal. At the very least, get a notepad or a calendar which has writing space.

# Week 1: Put It In Writing

| Sunday, Date *September 24* | | Planned | | Eaten | | Activities, Goals, Notes |
|---|---|---|---|---|---|---|
| Time | Food or Drink Item | Cal | Fat | Cal | Fat | |
| 8:00 | coffee, 1 Tbsp cream | | | 29 | 3 | did not sleep well |
| | bagel | | | 240 | 1 | |
| | 4 Tbsp cream cheese (2 oz) | | | 196 | 20 | 10am dentist appointment |
| 10:30 | M&Ms, 1.69 oz bag | | | 228 | 11 | |
| | | | | | | |
| 11:30 | Qtr pound cheeseburger | | | 510 | 28 | |
| | large order fries | | | 400 | 22 | |
| | 22 oz soda with ice | | | 260 | 0 | |
| 2:50 | potato chips, 1 oz | | | 150 | 10 | very tired, mild headache |
| | 12 oz soda | | | 155 | 0 | |
| 5:00 | (2) 12 ounce light beers | | | 224 | 0 | |
| | grilled chicken breast 4 oz | | | 187 | 4 | |
| | broccoli, 1 cup | | | 44 | 0 | |
| | garlic bread, 1 Tbsp butter | | | 175 | 12 | |
| 10:00 | 1 cup ice cream | | | 460 | 34 | |
| | | | | | | |
| | Total | | | 3258 | 145 | Weight: 220.5 |
| Monday, Date *September 25* | | | | | | |
| | | | | | | |
| | | | | | | |
| | | | | | | |
| | | | | | | |
| | | | | | | |
| | | | | | | |
| | | | | | | |
| | | | | | | |
| | | | | | | |
| | | | | | | |
| | | | | | | |
| | | | | | | |
| | | | | | | |
| | | | | | | |
| | | | | | | |
| | | | | | | |
| | | | | | | |
| | | | | | | |
| | | | | | | |
| | Total | | | | | Weight: |

Record what you eat *before* eating to make it a more conscious and deliberate act.

# Week 1: Put It In Writing

| Sunday, Date_____ | | Planned | | Eaten | | Activities, Goals, Notes |
|---|---|---|---|---|---|---|
| Time | Food or Drink Item | Cal | Fat | Cal | Fat | |
| | | | | | | |
| | | | | | | |
| | | | | | | |
| | | | | | | |
| | | | | | | |
| | | | | | | |
| | | | | | | |
| | | | | | | |
| | | | | | | |
| | | | | | | |
| | | | | | | |
| | | | | | | |
| | | | | | | |
| | | | | | | |
| | | | | | | |
| | | | | | | |
| | | | | | | |
| | | | | | | |
| | | | | | | |
| | | | | | | |
| | Total | | | | | Weight: |
| Monday, Date_____ | | | | | | |
| | | | | | | |
| | | | | | | |
| | | | | | | |
| | | | | | | |
| | | | | | | |
| | | | | | | |
| | | | | | | |
| | | | | | | |
| | | | | | | |
| | | | | | | |
| | | | | | | |
| | | | | | | |
| | | | | | | |
| | | | | | | |
| | | | | | | |
| | | | | | | |
| | | | | | | |
| | | | | | | |
| | | | | | | |
| | | | | | | |
| | Total | | | | | Weight: |

Record what you eat *before* eating to make it a more conscious and deliberate act.

- Weigh or measure portions until you are an expert at estimation. Get used to knowing the calorie and fat content of the foods you routinely eat. Record the time that you are eating, the number of calories (**cal**) and the fat grams (**fat**) that you consumed. Refer to the Sample Food Journal above. For now, leave the two columns of the Sample Journal Page under "Planned" blank. We will use these columns in Week 4.

- Be brutally honest in recording portions. Record each spoonful of dinner that you taste from the pots, every chocolate kiss that you grab from the office candy jar, every drink, meals and snacks. Do your best to estimate the amount of calories in everything you eat. Always err on the side of overestimation. This is not for your spouse, doctor, or friend to see. You can choose who sees it, or it can be for your eyes only. Do not be judgmental. Just record the facts as if you were recording data for a scientific experiment.

- Get a pocket calorie and fat guide which includes nutrition facts for common foods, brand name products and popular restaurant choices. Browse through the guide and compare the calories and fat content of many of your usual foods.

- Don't be tempted to rely on your memory. If your journal is too large or cumbersome to carry, get a tiny notepad and record the food items and quantity. You can then later calculate the fat and calories and transcribe this into your larger, more detailed journal in the evening. Keep your journal or notepad nearby always.

- It is vitally important that you record what you eat *before* you eat it. This will make the process of eating a more conscious and deliberate act. While calculating the calories that you are about to ingest, you will have the opportunity to choose not to eat, to eat less, or to make a better food choice. Recording the act also gives you an extra few seconds to consider the consequences.

- You can use your food journal to pinpoint any food related causes of energy level, mood fluctuation or allergies. If you are interested in this, each day record your mood or your allergy related symptom in the "Activities, Goals, Notes" section. Over time you may see patterns and correlations between what you eat and how you feel. Fatigue, headaches, irritability and many other symptoms can be caused by certain foods and relieved by diet changes. These symptoms will hinder your ability to stay on track and meet your goal. For an excellent reference on the impact of food on mood, see *Food & Mood* by Elizabeth Somer.

If, by the end of this week, you are not **accurately recording everything you eat and drink**, then start over again. Do this until it is second nature. At the end of the week review all your entries, but only for accuracy. Avoid being hard on yourself. You are not sup-

*Record what you eat before eating to make it a more conscious and deliberate act.*

posed to cut back this week. Your goal is to gain awareness of your eating habits, however poor they are, so you can begin the process of reshaping them into healthier habits. Throughout the remaining weeks of this year, we will work on turning those poor choices into healthier choices one by one. These early psychological changes will help you make this transition.

# Week 2: Breakfast of Champions

T here are 24 hours in one day, and those first few hours which include breakfast can set the pace for the whole day.

This week we will concentrate on the breakfast meal. At this point, continue to eat as you always have during the remainder of the day. Use your food journal to insure that you are not shifting the calories from the morning to other times of the day.

Breakfast is often overlooked as a problem meal. It can be a problem for three reasons:

1. Many people (especially dieters) tend to skip breakfast. However, this compounds hunger pains towards midday and the result is overeating for the rest of the day. Do not underestimate the importance of starting your day out right with a good breakfast. Your body needs fuel to start the day. Many studies have shown that a balanced breakfast results in greater productivity and concentration for workers, and better test scores for students.

2. Breakfast can also be a problem because the typical breakfast is high in fats, salt, sugar, calories and cholesterol: eggs, ham, bacon, pancakes, syrup, butter, hash browns, biscuits, sausage, hot chocolate, donuts and

sugar cereals. These are not only poor choices from a health standpoint, but they are also poor

> *I do not like green eggs and ham, I do not like them, Sam I Am! - Dr. Seuss*

choices for the time of day. The effect of these high-calorie foods will more likely send you right back to bed for a nap rather than jump-start your day.

3.  Because it is the first meal of the day, breakfast sets the stage for the rest of the day. If you start out the day with poor choices, you are more likely to finish out the day with more poor choices. On the other hand, a day started with a brisk walk and a sensible breakfast will be a constant reminder to lean towards better choices all day.

Take a close look at your typical breakfast and find where improvements can be made. Here are four different ways to reduce your intake of calories and fat during breakfast:

1.  Eat smaller portions. Have a half a bagel rather than a whole. Share the omelet with someone. Have one pancake, not three. Use a smaller cereal bowl and juice glass.

2.  Eat a full blown breakfast less often. Have your pancakes and syrup only once a month rather than twice a week.

3.  Choose better breakfast fare. This is the best alternative because you will be exchanging the traditional high-fat items for nutrient rich items. The best combination is a protein, starch and fruit. Protein will prevent mid-morning hunger. Choose fruit, cottage cheese, yogurt topped with a sprinkle of Grape Nuts, whole grain breads or cereals, juice, or a bowl of non-sugar cereal with skim milk. Avoid granolas which are usually high in fat and sugar. Rather than a croissant have a half bagel or

English muffin with jam. Oatmeal, Cream of Wheat or another warm cereal with a spoonful of brown sugar or honey can be wonderfully soothing and filling. There is also no reason why you need to eat traditional breakfast foods. A bowl of soup or leftover pasta is perfectly acceptable.

4. Choose a lighter variety of an item. Have your toast but spread with fresh preserves rather than butter. Try low-fat cream cheese on your bagel. Always use two egg whites to one egg yolk. Cook your french toast or eggs in a non-stick pan rather than fried in butter. Have a sprinkle of powdered sugar on your waffle instead of syrup. Better yet, top your waffle with blueberries. Have non-dairy, non-fat creamer in your coffee instead of cream. You probably won't taste a difference, and you can eliminate two to ten grams of fat per day.

Choose a combination of the above or whichever one works for you best. Starting this week, plan to have three breakfasts a week consisting of better choices. Make one of those days a weekend day. Write this in your journal, in the "Notes" section, as a reminder. After a few weeks, increase this to four, then five better breakfasts each week. Of course, you can jump right in and start with better breakfasts everyday. Just don't move so fast that you feel deprived or overly hungry.

Fast food can be tempting for breakfast, but is one of the worst choices. We are often in a hurry in the morning, and that fast food window is often all too easy. Most items on the fast food breakfast menu are loaded with fat. If time is your issue, work on ways to make breakfast easier. Have cold cereals, instant hot cereals, fruit, yogurt and low-fat cottage cheese in the refrigerator. Before you go to bed, decide what you'll eat for breakfast and do what you can to prepare the night before. Try to avoid a last minute choice. Having to choose when you are hungry and in a hurry often results in a poor choice.

Compare how you feel throughout the day on those days that you start with a healthy breakfast with the days you do not. You should have more energy and more incentive to continue the day on a healthy note. Remind yourself often during the day that you are moving close to your goal.

If you are not eating breakfast now, this is an excellent opportunity to start a new healthy habit. You can use breakfast to gain another fruit serving for the day. Yogurt with an apple or banana for breakfast will be a welcome addition to your diet.

Remember, it's not the once a month indulgence that keeps you overweight. It's consistent, multiple, poor choices over a long period of time. You don't have to let go of that favorite meal forever. Just modify, and get it under control. Then you can enjoy it even more.

# WEEK 3: WHAT'S YOUR DREAM?

This week, you will set your goal. Other than keeping your Food Journal and taking control of the breakfast hour, continue to eat as you always have. Many of the changes in these first weeks, such as this one, will realign your thinking towards your new lifestyle.

Goal setting has been proven time and time again to significantly increase the chances of success of any plan. Goals help you focus and keep you from drifting away from your original target.

> *Obstacles are those frightful things you see when you take your eyes off the goal.*
> *-Hannah More*

Successful goals are both *achievable* and *specific*. When formulating your goal, make sure that the end result is achievable. If you try to maintain a weight that keeps you starving, your body will not know how to regulate metabolism and appetite. It is unrealistic and probably unhealthy to aim for the figure of a model, or to aim for weight loss of more than a pound a week.

I was overweight for most of my teenage and young-adult years. After finally gaining control of my weight, I suffered for many months to maintain an "ideal" weight. I obsessed over every bite, every meal, every ounce gained or lost. I deprived myself of many favorite foods. I had worked hard to achieve that weight and wanted to maintain it. However, it soon became clear that I *never* felt satisfied, and was often preoccupied with the thought of the next meal. Food was still controlling my life. I also felt that I looked too thin in the face and neck, and had lost many of the curves in my figure. I eased up a bit, just a bit, and stabilized at about 10 pounds over my "ideal" weight. At this weight I feel great and my appetite is satisfied. I don't feel deprived or obsessed. My clothes fit great. My energy level is higher than ever. I've reached a most comfortable compromise—one that satisfies my appetite, my health and the reflection in the mirror.

You should feel comfortable with your weight—in your looks, health and appetite. Say your "weight chart" ideal is 115 pounds, but you now weigh 220. How would you feel at 140? Pretty good? Yes! If you can go lower without sacrificing taste and satisfaction, then do

> *Find a comfortable compromise—one that satisfies your appetite, your health and the reflection in the mirror.*

so. But if going lower means obsessing on every bite and choice, then you are still a prisoner of food and in danger of relapsing into old habits. If, after your body is completely adjusted to your new weight, you still wish to lose more, then make a few more minor adjustments in your eating habits.

So this week decide, realistically, what you want to weigh by the end of the year. You should not lose more than one pound a week. Your goals can be weekly, monthly, quarterly or for the entire year. If you have many pounds to lose, it may be better to target "one pound a week" rather than "65 pounds this year." After all, we are going to be chipping away at this problem ounce by ounce, day by day.

Use the following table as a guide to determine your goal weight.

## Suggested Healthy Weights For Adults

| Height* | Weight (lbs)**<br>Age 19-34<br>Years | Age 35 years<br>and over |
|---|---|---|
| 5'0" | ***97–128 | 108–138 |
| 5'1" | 101–132 | 111–143 |
| 5'2" | 104–137 | 115–148 |
| 5'3" | 107–141 | 119–152 |
| 5'4" | 111–146 | 122–157 |
| 5'5" | 114–150 | 126–162 |
| 5'6" | 118–155 | 130–167 |
| 5'7" | 121–160 | 134–172 |
| 5'8" | 125–164 | 138–178 |
| 5'9" | 129–169 | 142–183 |
| 5'10" | 132–174 | 146–188 |
| 5'11" | 136–179 | 151–194 |
| 6'0" | 140–184 | 155–199 |
| 6'1" | 144–189 | 159–205 |
| 6'2" | 148–195 | 164–210 |
| 6'3" | 152–200 | 168–216 |
| 6'4" | 156–205 | 173–222 |
| 6'5" | 160–211 | 177–228 |
| 6'6" | 164–216 | 182–234 |

* Without shoes
** Without clothes
*** The higher weights apply to people with more muscle and bone, such as many men.
Source: Report of the Dietary Guidelines Advisory Committee on the Dietary Guidelines for Americans, 1990.

Don't Diet—*Live It!*

Successful goals are also *specific.* Your goal must be measurable in definable terms. Use a specific time-frame and number of pounds and/or inches. Some examples of specific, achievable goals are:

- I will lose two pounds every month for two years.

- I will stick with the *Live It!* Plan for the entire year. By the end of the year, my diet will be based on the Food Guide Pyramid, and I will be exercising at least 30 minutes three times a week.

- In one year I will be 50 pounds lighter, my cholesterol will be 30% lower, and I will be exercising for 30 minutes at least three times a week.

Let others know what your goal is. Make a bet with someone, say for $100, that you will be successful in meeting your goal. Commit yourself to this success. It is not optional. You will not change your mind. This time success is possible and attainable.

It is important to give yourself continual reminders of your goal. Make it come alive. *Write it in each day of your food journal.* Memorize it. Recite it before each meal. Recite it when you are drifting off to sleep. Tape it to your bathroom mirror so that it is the first thing you see in the morning. Put it up on the refrigerator. Embroider it onto a pillow. Teach it to your toddler. Put it on your mouse pad or screen saver. Think of ways that you will see it several times a day. This will be your mission focus. You will say it over and over—and it will come true.

# WEEK 4: PLANNING

T he goal of this week is **to consciously *decide* what you are going to eat and not deviate from that plan**. If you decide to eat two donuts for breakfast, a double cheeseburger and fries for lunch, a pizza for dinner, four sodas and two bowls of ice cream, that is up to you. Just be sure that these were the foods that *you* decided on the day before. Avoid being judgmental. We are modifying an important thought process this week.

> *A man, a plan, a canal—Panama!*
> *- Traditional Palindrome*

You will learn to be in control of what you eat. *Planning brings control.* Do not underestimate the power and importance of the skills you are forming in these first few weeks. Your success depends on developing these long term habit and diet modifications.

Starting on Sunday evening write down everything you plan to eat the next day. Set aside a specific time every day that you will commit to planning. Record the calories and fat grams in the columns under "Planned" in your food journal. Be honest. Your aim is to *stick to your plan*. If you plan to eat only carrots and celery tomorrow, you are setting yourself up for failure. Your only aim this week is to plan what you will eat, not to diet or eat less or change your eating habits, other than those we have already discussed.

Be fairly accurate with the times that you record. If you record "candy bar" at ten o'clock, then eat that candy bar at ten o'clock, not earlier. Of course, if you eat less than you planned, that's even better. Just because you have planned a snack or extra portion does not mean you must eat it. This may sound obvious, but make a conscious determination whether or not you are hungry before you eat something. If you are not particularly hungry, or if the food is not especially appealing, then take this opportunity to decline. This is how success happens—grab it every chance you can.

Plan for weaknesses and temptations. If a holiday is coming in which you historically overeat, be prepared. Don't go to a party famished. Keep yourself nourished and decide what and how much you are going to eat at an event. If you plan to splurge, plan to eat lightly the day before and day after the event. Sometimes just realizing the cause of cravings will help you fight them. You'll learn more tips for dealing with special occasions in Week 34: Celebrate!.

While you plan your eating day (or week), build your grocery list and plan your shopping trips. Buy only what is on your grocery list. You'll soon find that you are also saving time and money by planning your meals.

Of course, there are times when life does not go according to plan. For instance, you are invited to a dinner, or you don't get to the grocery store as planned, or certain foods are on sale. You can accommodate for these deviations, but they should be few and far between, and the calories and fat grams should approximate that of the food you had planned to eat. If you deviate from what you planned, simply cross the item out and write in what you ate instead.

During the coming year you will slowly modify your eating plan so that your diet resembles the Food Guide Pyramid (we'll discuss this in Week 7.) We will work on various times of the day, meals, food groups, increasing your activity level, problem areas and behavior modification.

Consult the chart below to determine a healthy eating pattern based on the Food Guide Pyramid. This is what your daily diet should look like in about a year, with the help of the weekly habit changes.

## Sample Food Patterns for a Day at Three Calorie Levels

| 1,600 calories is about right for sedentary women and some older adults | 2,200 calories is about right for most children, teenage girls, active women, and many sedentary men. Women who are pregnant or breastfeeding may need somewhat more. | 2,800 calories is about right for teenage boys, many active men, and some very active women. |
|---|---|---|
| Calories | About 1,600 | About 2,200 | About 2,800 |
| Bread Servings | 6 | 9 | 11 |
| Fruit Servings | 2 | 3 | 4 |
| Vegetable Servings | 3 | 4 | 5 |
| Meat Group | 5 ounces | 6 ounces | 7 ounces |
| Milk Servings | 2-3* | 2-3* | 2-3* |
| Total Fat (grams)** | 53 | 73 | 93 |
| Total added sugars (teaspoons) | 6 | 12 | 18 |

*Women who are pregnant or breastfeeding, teenagers, and young adults to age 24 need three servings.

**Values for total fat and added sugars include fat and added sugars that are in food choices from the five major food groups as well as fat and added sugars from foods in the Fats, Oils, and Sweets group.

Source: Using The Food Guide Pyramid: A Resource for Nutrition Educators U.S. Department of Agriculture Food, Nutrition, and Consumer Services Center For Nutrition Policy and Promotion, 1995

Should you be counting fat, calories, or servings? Theoretically, if you count your servings and go strictly by the Food Guide Pyramid, there is no need to count calories or fat. However, sometimes it is difficult to decide which food group a particular food falls in. Since it is important to keep your fat intake to less than 30% of your total caloric intake, you should count both calories and fat. To make things very simple, use this rule: never eat (or buy) anything that has more than 30% of calories derived from fat. The total calories and the calories from fat are indicated on the Nutrition Facts label. If everything you eat consists of less than 30% calories derived from fat, then just counting calories will do.

Please note that the dietary and exercise guidelines in this book are appropriate for healthy adults. If you have a medical condition that requires specific dietary or activity level consideration, you should consult your doctor and/or registered dietitian before modifying your diet or activity level.

If, by the time this week is over, you are not accurately planning what you are eating, then start the week over. It is important that you have this habit completely established before you move on to the next weeks. As mentioned before, this week you do not have to modify your eating habits (other than breakfast). In fact, concentrate totally on the act of planning. This is how you will take control of your diet.

Consider your daily diet plan a promise to yourself. Be kind and honest with yourself and keep those promises.

# WEEK 5: THE MID-MORNING HOURS

T his week we will work on the tiny time slot between breakfast and lunch. You can still eat what you normally would at other times of the day. Eat a controlled breakfast. Then, plan to eat a snack that is less than 150 calories and less than three grams of fat during the time between breakfast and lunch. After lunch you can eat as you always have, but not more than usual!

Concentrate on one half hour increments. If you feel like snacking, remind yourself that you can have a snack that you prepared earlier, but put it off for one more half hour. Divert your attention from eating—go for a walk, take the stairs up and down two flights, make a phone call or read a magazine. The closer you can make it to lunch, all the better. In fact, if you eat your snack twenty minutes before lunch, your appetite for lunch will be reduced considerably.

If you have been overeating during this time period for years, this may be difficult for you. Your body may be expecting certain snacks at certain times. But stick with it—in about three to four weeks, this new habit will be firmly in place. Your body will adjust and will no longer send those hunger pains during this time period. Our bodies have wonderful internal alarms that you can regulate.

Don't Diet—*Live It!*

Just as you routinely wake up at a certain time, and become sleepy at about the same time every day, your body also becomes accustomed to eating at certain times of day. With persistence, you can change these clockwork cravings.

Check your journal during the week and make sure that you are not eating more in the afternoon to compensate for your reductions in the morning. Look back through the last

> *Curious things, habits. People themselves never knew they had them. –Agatha Christie*

weeks and count up how many extra calories you have been consuming during this time slot. You should be reducing your daily intake of calories by that amount. It may be only 100 or so calories, but reducing 100 calories each day adds up to a pound a month. And this is just the beginning. To make this easy, try these tips:

- Make your snacks for each day in the morning and put the correct portions in sandwich bags. Don't eat from the big bag. Take your snacks to work, so you won't be tempted by the snack machine. Leave your pocket change at home.

- Try hot snacks such as soups which are more satisfying and filling.

- Keep your snacks to under 150 calories and under three grams of fat.

Take a walk through your grocery store, read labels and compile a list of snacks that are appealing to you. The following are some snack ideas. Note that not all brands of each snack will contain the same number of calories and fat grams. For instance, a one-half cup serving of yogurt can vary from 70 to 250 calories and from 0 to 9 grams of fat. Compare several brands and flavors and keep your choices to those with under 150 calories and 3 grams of fat.

- Soup. Dried soups in-a-cup are great for work. Just fill with hot water from the coffee maker. Be sure to read the Nutrition Facts label, however, because some soups are packaged as two or three servings.

- A cup of unbuttered, air-popped popcorn sprinkled with dry Butter Buds, or any dry spice such as chili powder or popcorn seasoning.

- Three quarters to one cup cereal such as Cheerios, Shredded Wheat or Chex.

- A piece of bread or roll. Breads rich in whole grains will be tastier and more substantial than bread made with bleached white flour.

- An ounce of pretzels. Beware of the high sodium content of some pretzels.

- A rice cake. Rice cakes are now available in great flavors, from caramel to white cheddar.

- Sugar-free pudding or Jell-O. I limit my intake of artificial sweeteners, so this would be just an occasional snack. Make your pudding with skim or 1% milk.

- Non-fat (baked) or reduced fat potato chips. There are several brands and flavors available. Some are much better than others.

- Sugar-free yogurt topped with Grape Nuts.

- Melba toast and salsa.

- Low-fat cottage cheese with a slice of tomato or cantaloupe cubes.

- A piece of fresh fruit. The enormous variety of fruit can keep your snacks interesting for weeks.

- A serving of dried fruit such as raisins or pineapple.

- A serving of fruit canned in it's own juices.

- Applesauce with cinnamon.

- A cup of fruit juice. Beware of added sodium and sugars. Look for "100% fruit juice" on the label.

- Hot chocolate made with skim or 1% milk.

- Warm cereal such as grits, Cream-of-Wheat or oatmeal.

- Vegetables such as carrots, celery, cherry tomatoes and a yogurt based dip.

- Chinese chili-rice crackers.

- Non-fat fruit Newtons.

- Vanilla Wafers.

- A frozen fruit bar.

- A half-cup of sherbet.

- Graham crackers.

- A frozen fruit-yogurt bar.

- One half cup non-fat frozen yogurt.

If you normally eat something sweet, try yogurt or sugar-free pudding as a substitute. If you crave salty crunchy snacks, try pretzels instead of potato chips. It may be difficult to substitute your favorite snack. But just try it—eating a 150 calorie snack will take the edge off of your craving, and put it out of your mind. Then after you've made the right choice, you'll have the added satisfaction that you are gaining control of your eating habits.

Your ultimate goal is to eat three nutrient-rich meals a day, and two or three light snacks per day. You don't have to rush. You have plenty of time to move towards this in a controlled manner. By the end of the year you will be there—slowly, deliberately, and surely.

# WEEK 6: THE BUDDY SYSTEM

The reason that programs such as Weight Watchers and Alcoholics Anonymous work so well is that there is a wonderful support structure of people who share their goals and solutions. The support of two groups of people will help you: those who are not overweight, and those who also have a weight problem.

Hopefully, your family and friends who are not overweight will support you in your efforts. However, if they have not faced the challenges that you are facing, they may not understand the effort or rewards. They may not

> *It's so much more friendly with two.*
> *-Piglet, Pooh's Little Instruction*
> *Book, inspired by A. A. Milne*

even notice when you have lost an appreciable amount of weight. You may have to actually coach a close friend or family member to help you. Tell them that you are changing your life and their support is needed. Let them know that you have lost a few pounds and how good that feels. Invite them to celebrate with you. Ask them how they might best help you. Perhaps they can help you plan your eating day. Also, ask them for help when you feel down or losing control.

The other group of people, those with similar weight problems, are an important part of your support structure for two reasons: to help you reach your goals and *more importantly, to lend your strength in helping them meet theirs.*

You may question your strength, but if you have come this far, you have demonstrated strength of commitment. You have something to give. Why is it more important to help someone else?

*The best way to cheer yourself up is to try to cheer somebody else up.*
*-Mark Twain*

In addition to being benevolent, you help yourself even more if you focus on helping someone else. You will raise your self esteem and take the focus away from your problems. If you obsess on your failures or seek support simply to help yourself, then you are still controlled by the issues that contributed to your weight. Lending your strength will make you even stronger.

You can learn from others and you can help others reach their goals. You can draw from another's strengths. You can share ideas. You can help each other focus. Having a partner doubles your initiative. You may be low on self-discipline one day, but chances are your partner is not, and he can help you through that weak time. Another person can inspire, offer encouragement and support. And you can do the same for them.

You of course must find an individual who is ready to make a change. Use your enthusiasm to help them start. Share a copy of the *Live It!* Plan with them. If you have a family member or friend who is overweight but not willing or ready to change, you cannot and should not force your new lifestyle on them, but you can be a living example of how good eating can turn your life around. Use a silent but powerful, example-setting approach.

Losing weight with your spouse can be ideal. You'll both eat the same meals and look forward to similar goals. You can participate in the same activities. However, if you are a woman, and your support partner is a man, be aware that he will probably lose weight quicker, and he will probably have more strength while exercising.

*Keep your fears to yourself, but share your courage with others.*
*- Robert Louis Stevenson*

This may be frustrating unless you realize that the weight loss is relative. Choose activities that you can both enjoy at your individual paces. You may not be able to compete with a man in tennis, but you certainly can enjoy a canoe trip or hike together.

Your support structure may be down the street, in your own home, a weekly phone call, email correspondences, on the Internet, or at a local weight control group. You can start your own neighborhood support group. Just have a meeting once a week. Share ideas, recipes and motivation. Find a group that works for you and one where you can make a contribution. Spend the week building this support structure and make the commitment to stick with it. Someone out there needs you.

# WEEK 7: GET THE SKINNY

T his week you will build a foundation of information that will help you make healthy decisions for the rest of your life. Even if you think you already know these facts, spend this week becoming an expert. Your goal this week is to **develop a habit of consciously thinking about the nutritional content of everything you eat**. It's true—you are what you eat. You've already started this process by recording what you eat, but now we will take it a step further.

*Avoid fruits and nuts.*
*You are what you eat.*
*-Jim Davis (Garfield the Cat)*

Knowing what you are eating has never been so easy. The Nutrition Labeling and Education Act of 1990 (NLEA) was enacted to provide mandatory nutrition labeling of all foods by May 1994. The guidelines make it easier to compare foods and to see how certain foods fit into your daily eating plan.

Obviously, to reach your weight goal, you must make changes in the way that you eat and in your activity level. The Dietary Guidelines for Americans, developed in 1995 by the Department of Health and Human Services and the U.S. Department of Agriculture are:

**1. Eat a variety of foods** to get the nutrients that you need for good health. Your body needs about 50 different nutrients every day, and no one or two foods contains all these nutrients. Choose foods within and across the basic five food groups in the Food Guide Pyramid (see an illustration of the Food Guide Pyramid in Appendix A.) Follow the guidelines for the number of servings from each group, and vary your selections within each group.

**2. Balance the food you eat with physical activity—** maintain or improve your weight. You should accumulate 30 minutes or more of moderate physical activity on most, preferably all, days of the week. Brisk walking, jogging, swimming, housework, dancing and gardening are examples of moderate activity. We will phase in activity in Weeks 9, 20, 33 and 46.

**3. Eat a diet with plenty of grain products, vegetables and fruit.** Your meals should be centered around a grain food such as rice, pasta or bread. Fruits and vegetables should make up the next largest portion of your diet. Foods from these groups will be naturally lower in fat and calories than food from the meat and fat group. They will also provide essential nutrients required for a healthy diet. Most Americans do not eat the recommended number of servings of grain products, vegetables and fruits, resulting in a diet that is too high in fats, sugar and sodium. Weeks 16, 22, 28, and 41 focus on ways to get more grain products, fruits and vegetables in your diet.

**4. Choose a diet low in fat, saturated fat, and cholesterol—**your diet should consist of no more than 30 percent of calories from fat, or about 65 grams of fat in a 2,000 calorie daily diet; and no more than ten percent of calories, or 20 grams of fat, from saturated fats. Ounce for ounce, fats contain more than twice as many calories as carbohydrates or proteins.

It is important to note that this is a *percent of calories*, not *percent fat*. Be sure to look at the Nutrition Facts label. The **Calories from Fat** should be one-third of the total **Calories**.

Many of the habits and tips that you will learn this year will either directly or indirectly result in a reduced intake of fats. Weeks 11, 24, 42 and 45 specifically help you reduce your intake of fats, especially saturated fats.

**5. Choose a diet moderate in sugars.** Highly refined sugars are concentrated calories with sparse nutrients. Your teeth, as well as your weight, will benefit from reduced sugar. Week 32 addresses this issue.

**6. Choose a diet moderate in salt and sodium.** Sodium, or salt, occurs naturally in foods, and usually in small amounts. Most of the sodium that we ingest comes from prepared and processed foods. Sodium promotes water retention and is associated with higher blood pressure. High salt intake also increases the amount of calcium that is excreted in urine, which increases the body's need for calcium.

Following the Food Guide Pyramid recommendations of eating plenty of fruits and vegetables will naturally lower your intake of sodium. Week 25 is devoted to reducing sodium levels.

**7. If you drink alcoholic beverages, do so in moderation**— the maximum alcohol consumption should be about one drink a day for women, two for men. Alcohol contains calories but few or no nutrients. Alcohol can alter your judgment and lessen your resolve to stick to your goal.

During this entire week, establish a habit to look at the nutritional content of the foods you eat. Become familiar with the Nutrition Facts labeling. Learn what a "portion" is. It is helpful to equate a portion of something with a reference. For instance, a four ounce portion of meat, cut one quarter inch thick, is approximately equal in size to your palm (if your hand is of medium size.)

As you look at product claims, know that there are certain terms that, by law, can only be used to describe food products with certain qualities. A table with these terms follows.

## Food Product Claims

| Term | Can be used to describe a product that |
|---|---|
| Low-fat | contains three grams or less per serving |
| Low-saturated fat | contains one gram or less per serving |
| Low-sodium | contains 140 mg or less per serving |
| Very low sodium | contains 35 mg or less per serving |
| Low-cholesterol | contains 20 mg or less and two grams or less of saturated fat per serving |
| Low-calorie | contains 40 calories or less per serving. |
| Lean | is meat, poultry, or seafood with less than 10 g fat, 4.5 g or less saturated fat, and less than 95 mg cholesterol per serving and per 100 g. |
| Extra lean | is meat, poultry, seafood, and game meats with less than five g fat, less than two g saturated fat, and less than 95 mg cholesterol per serving and per 100 g |
| High | contains 20% or more of the Daily Value for a particular nutrient in a serving. |
| Good source | contains 10 to 19% of the Daily Value for a particular nutrient in one serving. |
| Reduced | is a nutritionally altered product that contains at least 25% less of a nutrient or of calories than the regular, or reference, product. |
| Less | contains 25% less of a nutrient or of calories than the reference food. For example, pretzels that have 25% less fat than potato chips could carry a "less" claim. "Fewer" is an acceptable synonym. |
| Light | 1. is a nutritionally altered product that contains one-third fewer calories or half the fat of the reference food. If the food derives 50% or more of its calories from fat, the reduction must be 50% of the fat, OR2. is a low-calorie, low-fat food that has 50% less sodium. "light in sodium" may describe food in which the sodium content has been reduced by at least 50%, OR3. is light in texture, color, or another property as long as the label explains the intent-for example, "light brown sugar" and "light and fluffy." |
| More | contains a nutrient that is at least 10% of the Daily Value more than the reference food in one serving |
| Healthy | is low in fat and saturated fat and has limited amounts of cholesterol and sodium. Also, if it's a single-food item, it must provide at least 10% of one or more of vitamins A or C, iron, calcium, protein or fiber. If it's a meal type product, it must provide 10% of two or three of those items in addition to meeting other criteria. |
| Percent fat-free | that is a low-fat or a fat-free. In addition, the claim must accurately reflect the amount of fat present in 100 g of the food. Thus, if a food contains 2.5 g fat per 50 g, the claim must be "95% fat-free." |

Get more information from the library, your healthcare professional and health publications. A terrific source of current research on nutrition is the *Nutrition Action Health Letter* from the Center for Science in the Public Interest. This well-researched monthly newsletter does not hesitate to expose food manufacturers that make misleading claims on their products. Your medical doctor's office and/or insurance company should also be able to provide information on nutrition. Many insurance programs will even provide nutrition classes. Your local public health clinic, the Department of Health and Human Services and the U.S. Department of Agriculture are also good sources of information.

> *Get the facts first. You can distort them later.*
> *- Mark Twain*

A less conventional source of information will be your local health food store. Most will have a well stocked bookshelf, and will sponsor lectures by various nutrition experts. In addition to publications related to mainstream research, you'll find alternative theories. Keep yourself well informed and be sure that the theories that you subscribe to are based in solid, accurate and recent research. See Appendix C: Bibliography and Appendix D: Internet Sites of Interest for an excellent list of references.

The Food Guide Pyramid is probably far, far from how you actually eat now. Don't be discouraged. Just as you should not be judging yourself when you record what you eat, do not judge these guidelines now. Simply learn them. Plant a seed. By the end of the year, you will have *painlessly* moved into this model. It is achievable, and yes, you can have a healthy *and* satisfying diet. You won't know what hit you.

# WEEK 8: THE WATER WAY

C ontrolling your weight includes much more than reducing calories and increasing activity. One subtle but important element in weight control and health is water. This week, continue to follow the guidelines of the previous weeks and start drinking at least **64 ounces of water a day**. If you are outside during a hot day or more active than usual, you should drink even more.

You should drink consistently throughout the day. If you wait until you are thirsty, your body is already dehydrated. Drinking plenty of water is vital to weight control has many healthy benefits:

- Aids in the digestion of food and absorption of nutrients.

- Reduces constipation. Helps food move through the digestive tract.

- Reduces water retention. If you don't drink enough water, you body will tend to retain water as it would in a drought. Give it the water that it needs, and it won't retain.

- Improves the appearance and feel of skin and hair.

- Reduces your thirst which otherwise may be quenched with a high-calorie drink such as a cola or beer.

Get in the habit of taking a quart of water for extended car trips and always while exercising. Find a leak proof sport bottle and always keep it filled and close at hand. Find one that is convenient, easy to hold, easy to fill, easy to drink from and one that you will want to use. If you walk, jog or bike, find a bottle you can strap on. If a sports bottle does not appeal to you, find a great crystal glass or mug that you'll *want* to drink from.

Note that water means *water*. Not colas, beer, juice, coffee or tea. You certainly do not want to start a new bad habit or add unnecessary and empty calories to your diet for the sake of hydration. Caffeine and alcohol can deplete vitamins and can actually cause you to de-

> *I went on a diet, swore off drinking and heavy eating, and in fourteen days I lost two weeks.*
> *– Joe E. Lewis*

hydrate. Even though fruit juice has many nutrients, it is also high in calories and should be considered a fruit serving.

Should you drink tap water, filtered water or bottled water? This is a surprisingly complicated question. Drinking a variety of waters can be important. Tap water is always available, virtually free and there's no container to throw away. However, tap water, either from a well or municipal water treatment plant, may contain contaminants which can be harmful if ingested in large quantities. Contaminants can come from the treatment plant, your well, the path that the water takes to your house, or your household pipes and faucets. These contaminants can be naturally occurring, from human or animal waste, or from industrial waste. Health risks include cancer, damage to vital organs, nervous system damage and gastrointestinal diseases. Since you will be drinking a large amount of water, choosing your water sources can be important. You can choose from a variety of filters that can remove many contaminants from tap water. No filter removes all contaminants. Boiling can kill microorganisms, but will also concentrate harmful chemicals. If you are concerned about a particular contaminant, you can have your water tested and then seek a filter that removes that contaminant. Your state government should be able to provide you with information on the possible contaminants in your area, and water testing labs. Here are some sources of more information on safe drinking water:

- EPA (Environmental Protection Agency) regulates municipal water sources. The EPA issued the Safe Drinking Water Act Amendments of 1996. A publication for consumers describing this legislation can be ordered from the EPA at (800)426-4791. This publication also lists other resources on safe drinking water. You can also visit the EPA website at www.epa.gov.

- FDA (Food and Drug Administration) regulates bottled water as a food product. Their website is www.fda.gov.

- The IBWA (International Bottled Water Association) is a self-governing trade association which represents the bottled water industry. You can request a free publication which answers questions about bottled water regulations by calling (800)928-3711.

- The NSF (National Sanitation Foundation) is a non-profit organization that tests and certifies bottled water, water additives, water filtration and purification systems. You can obtain a consumer book listing water filters and bottled waters by calling (800)673-6275. There is a $6 shipping and handling fee. The NSF maintains a very informative website where you can search the product database and find filters and bottled waters that remove specific contaminants. This site, www.nsf.org, is well-worth a visit.

Certainly in some areas of the world, bottled or filtered water will taste better. The water source you choose will be your personal preference. Experiment and find a few that are pleasant. A squeeze of fresh lemon or lime in your water can make a tremendous difference in the taste. After a short time, you will prefer water to quench your thirst over flavored beverages.

If drinking cold water all day gives you a chill, try warm or even hot water. Hot water (the same temperature as coffee or hot tea) can be very soothing. A hot drink can also give you a feeling of fullness and contentment and take the edge off of hunger between meals.

Devise a way to remind yourself throughout the day to drink. One way to keep track of the amount of water you drink is to fill a half gallon container each morning. Leave it on the kitchen counter as a reminder and pour your water from this jug. The jug should be empty by the end of the day. Or put eight pennies or buttons in your pocket. Each time you drink one eight ounce glass of water, move a penny to the opposite pocket.

Drinking water is a habit that is easy to adopt and one that can make a big difference in your health.

# WEEK 9: GET THE LEAD OUT

Y es, all successful weight management plans include ways to expend more calories than you consume. In addition to losing weight by burning calories, exercise will help you to:

- Lose fat
- Build muscle
- Improve your overall health including lowered blood pressure and reduced risk of osteoporosis
- Increase your overall strength and endurance
- Digest your food
- Help you sleep better
- Control your appetite
- Release endorphins which make you feel good
- Reduce stress
- Increase your metabolism
- Avoid boredom which can trigger over-eating

The evidence is overwhelming that exercise is vital to maintaining a healthy body. But this doesn't have to mean a boring jogging routine or embarrassing session at the gym. Rather than submitting yourself to a rigid exercise schedule, adopt two infinitely less painful, and even satisfying ways to become more active:

> *A bear, however hard he tries,*
> *grows tubby without exercise.*
> *-Pooh's Little Instruction Book,*
> *inspired by A. A. Milne*

1. This week, we focus on becoming more active during ordinary everyday activities.

2. Next quarter, you will choose activities that you look forward to and that have benefits in addition to losing weight.

Recent studies indicate that it is not necessary to perform your exercise in one daily session. Activity spread throughout the day can be just as effective. All of the following activities can be done without joining a gym, getting a baby-sitter, buying equipment, taking a shower afterwards, or by setting aside blocks of time of your day. Many can be done with a friend, spouse, pet, neighbor or child. Some good examples are:

- Parking an extra 20 cars away *every* time you park can add up to 4.5 miles per month. How? Twenty parking spaces is about 200 feet. Walk into and out of work and into and out of one store and that equals 800 feet per day. In 30 days you've walked 24,000 feet, or about 4.5 miles. And it was painless. No dread. No sweat. Fewer dings on your car. And you've left those closer spaces for the elderly, mothers with small children, and those feeling under the weather. Don't have time to park far away? I bet you spend more time prowling for a closer space than you would walking the distance.

- Sell or swap your power or riding mower for a non-powered mower. I had a neighbor who would cut his large lawn with a riding mower while drinking beer, then go to the gym for exercise. Never made much sense to me.

- Give away your leaf blower. Save yourself some money and get some great exercise at the same time. Eliminate the gas fumes and deafening sound. Use an old fashioned rake. Take in the sunshine, fresh air and sounds of the outdoors.

- Always return your grocery cart to the store. All the way.

- Get up every hour and perform a few minutes of exercise. Vacuum a room. Walk up and down stairs. Take a brisk walk around your block. This will revive you all day long. Set an alarm or a timer as a reminder. Five minutes of brisk exercise each hour for eight hours adds up to forty minutes.

- Every time you go to the restroom or water fountain, go to one on another floor, or take the long route to and from.

- Pick up your step! Walk, stand and sit straight and tall. Tone all your muscles. *Feel* your muscles when you move. Tuck your belly and bottom in. As you increase the distance you walk, also increase the speed. Swing your arms. Get the most out of every step. You'll not only look better, you'll use more calories and tone your muscles. Keep your head up. Look people in the eyes, and smile.

- Walk briskly around the office while waiting on the microwave.

- Don't use the remote control. Get up and adjust the TV.

Don't Diet—*Live It!*

- Swap thirty minutes of TV time for thirty minutes of household or yard chores every day. Just think of how much you could get done with an extra thirty minutes every day.

- Take your baby or toddler (or grandchild) to the park. Swing in the swings with them or catch and throw a ball.

- Rock in a rocking chair when watching TV.

- Put your waste basket outside of your office.

- Take the stairs instead of an elevator, and don't hesitate to run upstairs at home several times a day. Instead of putting an item on the stairs to be carried up, take it up right then.

- Get off the bus or train one stop before your usual.

- If you watch TV, mute the commercials and finish some housework. This can easily add up to ten minutes per hour.

- Offer to help a friend move.

- Are you often involved in long, seated meetings? Don't hesitate to get up every half and hour and stretch. Suggest a quick break for all. Move your legs. Change position often.

- Walk to see a neighbor or co-worker instead of phoning.

You get the picture. Increase the time that you are up and on you feet all day long. It really counts. Rather than face a 30 or 60 minute workout, you can split that time into smaller increments and get the same results. And there's no need to change clothes, get special equipment, or take a shower. You will be amazed at how soon some of these become habits and second nature. Limit the time during the day that you are idle. Get fidgety and *move!*

# WEEK 10: RATE YOUR WEIGHT

Now it's time to start a baseline for measuring your progress. Weight management experts disagree on how often to weigh or even what factors to use in tracking weight management. Body fat content, hip to waist ratio, inches, and weight can all be used to measure progress. We will use weight because it is easily measured and understood by most people.

You may prefer to weigh once a week rather than daily. Weighing daily can be discouraging and misleading. Even though you are losing fat, fluctuations in water retention or constipation can add weight. Increased activity produces sore muscles which take on water to heal. This means that you not only will weigh a bit more, but those sore muscles will swell a bit and you may feel thicker. Be aware of this so that you are not discouraged. The swelling will decrease, and you will be left with healthier, shapely, toned muscles and reduced fat.

Many other factors induce temporary water weight: hormonal changes, some drugs, sunburn, foods high in sodium, high starch meals, and not routinely drinking enough water. Some recent popular diets that are high in protein and low in carbohydrates will produce quick weight loss, but the loss is mainly water weight.

Don't Diet—*Live It!*

These diets can be very misleading and disappointing for those whose goal is lifelong weight control.

Also, muscle weighs more than fat and as you slim down your fat to muscle ratio will decrease significantly, especially if you are exercising. Two people can be the same height and size, but the one with more muscle mass will weigh more. So, you may be losing inches by replacing fat with muscle, but you may not lose as much weight as you expected. If you wish to weigh daily, be aware of these fluctuations in weight and do not let them discourage you.

Because your weight loss will be gradual (but deliberate and permanent), I recommend that you weigh only once a week. Always weigh at the same time of day, with the same amount of clothing (preferably none.) The best time is in the morning before eating or drinking anything. If you weigh once a week, do so on the same day of the week. Your weekday eating habits are probably different than your weekend habits, and your weight will fluctuate accordingly.

See the Sample Quarterly Weight Chart below. There is also a blank Weight Chart that you can photocopy for each quarter of the year. To use the Weight Chart, put your current weight in the upper left box of the chart. If you plan to lose one pound a week, subtract one pound and record that number in the box below your current weight. Continue subtracting one pound until you reach the bottom of the column. If you have a digital scale, you can even use one-half or one-tenth pound increments.

Highlight a diagonal line, using a bright color such as red or yellow, from your weight now on the upper left, to your goal weight for the end of the quarter on the lower right, just above week thirteen. This line will be your target. Your weight on some weeks may be above or below the line, but the general trend when followed over several weeks should follow the line. Try not to obsess about fractions of a pound. Tape the chart to your wall or keep it near your scale with a pencil.

Each time you weigh, plot a dot where your weight falls on the chart above the week. As the weeks progress, you can adjust your diet according to your rate of weight loss.

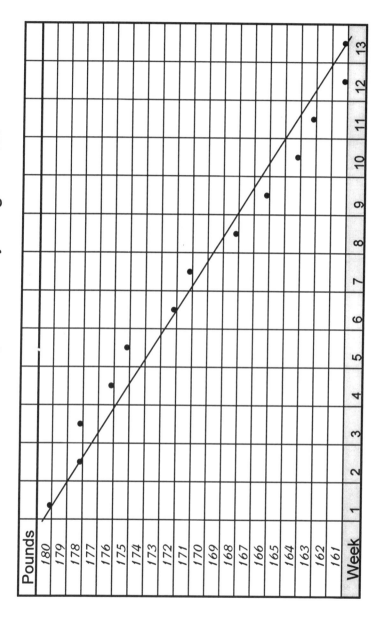

Sample Quarterly Weight Chart

# Quarterly Weight Chart

| Pounds | | | | | | | | | | | | | |
|---|---|---|---|---|---|---|---|---|---|---|---|---|---|
| Week | 1 | 2 | 3 | 4 | 5 | 6 | 7 | 8 | 9 | 10 | 11 | 12 | 13 |

# WEEK 11: DAIRY DON'TS

D airy products and eggs can account for a high percentage of fat, especially saturated fat, in the average diet. Though nutritious and a valuable source of vitamins and calcium, they can be needlessly high in calories and saturated fats.

Fats contain both saturated and unsaturated fatty acids. Saturated fats raise blood cholesterol levels more than unsaturated fats. Fats from animal products (meats, eggs and dairy products) are the main source of saturated fat in the typical diet. This type of fat should be limited to 20 grams in a 2,000 calorie per day diet. Although a small amount of fat is essential to the human diet, high-fat diets can lead to obesity, heart disease and some forms of cancer.

Olive oil and canola oil are particularly high in unsaturated fats. Other vegetable oils and fats from fish and nuts are good sources of unsaturated fats. These types of fats reduce blood cholesterol *when they replace* saturated fats in the diet. Unsaturated fats should make up most of the 65 grams of fat allowed in a 2,000 calorie diet.

Another type of unsaturated fat, trans-fatty acid, which is found in solid fats such as margarine and shortening, may raise blood cholesterol. As a general rule, you should avoid solid fats.

There are several ways to reduce the fat but still enjoy the taste and nutrients from dairy products. We will work on this task this week, and once again in the fourth quarter. Here's how to start:

- If you are now using whole milk, gradually move to skim. Start with 2% now. In your food journal, two months from now remind yourself to switch to 1%, then in another month to ½%, then skim. By the time you have adjusted to skim milk, you will not be able to stand the thick and fatty taste of whole milk. Always use skim milk for cooking items such as mashed potatoes, puddings and sauces. If you need a thickener, use arrow root and/or canned condensed skim milk. You will still get the nutrients of milk, but without the fat.

- Experiment with lower fat cheeses. Mozzarella from part-skim milk is an excellent substitute for the higher fat provolone, even melted in baked dishes. When using low-fat cheeses, follow the package directions regarding baking. Most will not melt well at high temperatures, but are quite acceptable when baked at lower temperatures. Many low-fat or fat-free cheeses are terrific when served cold. You may not be able to tell the difference. Try the reduced fat versions of ricotta and cream cheese. Substitute low-fat cottage cheese for ricotta in baked dishes. Try gradually mixing in the lower fat variety with the real thing. Your taste will adjust to the reduced fat content, just as it will with reduced fat milk.

- Substitute unflavored yogurt for sour cream as a base for a dip. Here again, you can try mixing yogurt and sour cream and slowly decrease the amount of sour cream over a period of weeks or months.

- Rather than whipping cream, try one of the light frozen or canned whipped creams, or non-dairy whipped topping, or marshmallow cream topping. Even though you are reducing fat, be sure to watch the calories. Many "low-fat" items are still quite high in sugar and calories.

- When using eggs, use one whole egg and only the white of another. All of the fat in an egg is in the yolk. If you make egg salad, use twice as many whites. This works great in omelets and french toast. Two whole eggs have 156 calories and ten grams of fat, but one whole egg plus two egg whites has 95 calories and only five grams fat. Egg whites can be whipped to increase their volume and make an omelet (or waffle batter) light and fluffy. As a general rule, you should limit your intake of egg yolks to two per week.

- Experiment with egg substitutes. They may or may not be suitable in every recipe, or for every taste. As you may have noticed, I rarely recommend using "fake" substitutes. I avoid the new "fake" fats, and rarely use sugar substitutes. Moderation can enable you to eat anything, and keeps taste and diversity in your diet.

Avoid introducing all of these tips at once. Rather, plant these tips in your food journal over the next several months. Try to adopt as many as you are comfortable with.

# WEEK 12: SET THE STAGE FOR SUCCESS

Keeping healthy eating habits can be tough in our consumer world. Temptations are everywhere, fueled by multi-billion dollar marketing budgets, but you can control the impact significantly. Devote this week to modifying your environment to give yourself the best possible chance for success. Here are some ideas:

- Once a week, after a good meal, take a visual inventory of your pantry and refrigerator. Don't hesitate to throw out an unhealthy item or two. Yes, it is hard to throw food away. Remind yourself the next time you buy it that the waste occurs when you *buy* it, not when you throw it away. Rather than thinking that this is a waste of money, consider how many years of your life you have been overweight and years you can lose due to poor health. Just throw it out. It won't help starving people across the globe if *you* eat it. If that is your concern, then buy less and donate the savings to a charity. This exercise will also make it easier for you to leave those last few bites on your plate when you have eaten enough.

- Put leftovers in serving size portions in the freezer. Put cheese, meats and snacks in the freezer. Don't leave any food out on the counters. Put your snacks in containers that are not transparent.

- Each day, prepare your two snacks and your lunch beforehand. A carefully prepared lunch is much safer than going through a cafeteria line, or deciding on what or where to eat when you are hungry. If you've prepared a good lunch that morning, then each time you think about lunch you will anticipate eating what you prepared. You will be less likely to be tempted by a spur of the moment craving. You can reach for pretzels in your desk drawer instead of potato chips in the snack machine.

- Leave the room during television commercials. Get a little bit of exercise during this time. This way, you will miss those snack and fast food commercials while you complete some housework or chores.

- Keep food in the kitchen only.

- Do you hit the snack machine often? If so, make sure that you do not carry change. Leave your change at home. Save it and splurge on a non-food fun item for every five pounds you lose.

- Lose the phone number for the local pizza delivery place. Don't clip coupons for unhealthy snacks and meals.

- Is there a donut club at the office? Move your desk or move the location of the donuts. Take your name off of the list and don't participate. Or, on your day, bring in fresh bagels instead.

An important step in modifying your environment is to separate the act of eating from your other activities. Never eat while doing something else such as reading, watching TV, or driving. Avoid eating in places such as your bedroom, your office, or your car. Eat only in your kitchen at home, or other places specifically designated for dining. Here are three compelling reasons for separating eating from other activities:

- Your food will not be as enjoyable if you are concentrating on something else. Wait until you can focus your attention on eating. Think about and savor every bite.

- If you eat while concentrating on something else, you will eat without realizing how much you are eating. Remember, eating should be a controlled and conscious act.

- Once you limit the *places* you eat, you will also limit the *times* you can eat. Your body will adjust to this so that you no longer have cravings when watching TV or when driving home from work.

There are other benefits to limiting eating to specific areas. Your car won't smell like french fries, you'll have less trouble with pests such as ants, roaches and rodents, and cleanup is much easier—no more crumbs in the sofa and no more drink stains on the carpet.

> *Cultivate only the habits that you are willing should master you.*
> *-Elbert Hubbard*

Everyone's environment and temptations are unique. Analyze yours. Where are your biggest temptations? Identify ten things you can do to remove temptation and improve your chances for success. Write these ten things down in your food journal and implement them one by one over the next few months.

# WEEK 13: FIRST QUARTER REVIEW

T ake this week to reflect, review, revise, reward, relax and recommit to your goal. You've come a long way. Do not be discouraged if you have not lost much weight. This quarter was important for laying a foundation for the next three quarters, and for the rest of your life. Skim back over the last thirteen weeks and review the aim for each week. Do one small thing during this week to reinforce the goal of each of the previous weeks such as:

*Put It In Writing:* Review how you kept your journal. Are you estimating portions correctly? Can you see a difference in your eating patterns since the first week? Are you moving in the right direction?

*Breakfast of Champions:* Make your next omelet with two egg whites and one yolk. Whip the whites a bit, then fold in the yolk. Cook in a non-stick skillet. Fill with diced tomatoes and peppers, or salsa. Sprinkle with non-fat shredded cheddar cheese.

*What's Your Dream?:* Is your goal realistic? Do you need to revise it? Have a mug made with your goal written on it.

*Planning:* Look at your menu plans critically and see how you can change them to gradually move towards the Food Guide Pyramid model.

*The Mid-Morning Hours:* Look through the grocery store and pick three more low-calorie snacks that you can have in the house or take to work.

*The Buddy System:* Touch base with your support structure. Let them help you with this review. How are they doing with their goal? Help them along also.

*Get the Skinny:* Read a current book on nutrition. Browse the book section in a health food store.

*The Water Way:* Buy yourself a great glass, mug or cup that you'll use only for water.

*Get the Lead Out:* Take the dog for a walk everyday. Don't have a dog? Borrow your neighbor's dog.

*Rate Your Weight:* Buy a better weight scale. A digital scale can have increments of a tenth of a pound which will make slow weight loss more detectable.

*Dairy Don'ts:* Rather than baking a pudding pie, bake pudding tarts: rather than a traditional crust using shortening, buy ready-made graham cracker crust tart shells. Fill with pudding made with skim or 1% milk, and top with reduced-fat whipped topping instead of whipped cream.

**Set the Stage for Success:** Drop your subscription to that food magazine, and get one that is geared towards healthy living such as light cooking, sports, crafts or travel. That monthly magazine in the mailbox is a great reminder to stay on track.

Give yourself a reward, even for a tiny improvement. If you wanted to lose twelve pounds but only lost four, that's still great! The most important thing is that you have *lost* and not *gained* and you are still committed to change. You have

> *If I'd known I was going to live this long, I'd have taken better care of myself.*
> *-Eubie Blake*

formed many habits that will produce terrific, lifelong results. In the next three months, you will move closer to the Food Guide Pyramid and see more results. You will build ways to change your focus from food to a focus on life, activity and health.

# SECOND

# QUARTER:

# FRAMEWORK

# BUILDING

# WEEK 14: MAKE IT LAST

T his week, you will lengthen the time it takes you to eat. Your goal is to *eat slowly*. It takes twenty minutes for food to metabolize sufficiently to send signals to your brain that turn off hunger. If you eat too fast you will over–eat by the time your brain turns off your appetite. This is a simple concept but one that works. By eating slowly you will also enjoy your food more while giving your body time to register fullness.

It is a natural tendency to eat fast. Our ancestors had to eat fast because they were in competition at the feast, both from other humans in the clan and from other predators. Remind yourself that deprivation is not a fact of life today in our country. You don't have to compete for food and it is readily available. Be thankful that you are not faced with the opposite problem—famine and starvation. Your challenge is to keep from being *over-nourished*. This is an intellectual challenge that few on this planet are lucky enough to face. It is also a challenge that you can meet with skills and knowledge.

Here are several tips to increase the time it takes to eat your meal:

- Increase the number of times you chew each bite. For instance, if you normally chew a piece of apple three times, increase to four or five times.

- Decide how long it will take you to eat your meal. Stick to that time frame.

- Think about each bite. *Taste* it. The longer it takes you to eat, the longer you can enjoy your food. Savor your food.

- Take smaller bites. Use a smaller fork or spoon. Cut your food into smaller portions.

- Take a bite, then put your fork down. Then take a drink of water. Ask yourself, after *each* bite, "Am I still hungry? Does this still taste as good as the first bite?"

- Mid way through the meal, stop and wait for two full minutes. Get up and put the leftovers away. Get another glass of water. Then sit down and reconsider whether you are still hungry, or whether you are eating simply because it is on your plate. This is a particularly effective tip. Try it.

- Eat your meal in courses. Start with a salad, vegetable, soup or bread before the main meal is finished cooking. Put away those dishes, put the leftovers away and then move on to the main course. This is also a great way to get your vegetables before you fill up on the less nutritious and more fattening main course.

- Use all your senses—smell your food, prepare a great looking plate with many colors and textures, and enjoy this as much as the taste.

- Look up and around during your meal. Avoid a head-down shoveling approach to eating.

Practice this until you have changed your eating pace. Time yourself. You will probably be surprised how quickly you can put away 3,000 calories. How many times have you over-eaten, and then fifteen minutes later thought "Why did I eat so much?" When this happens, when you over-indulge, learn from it. Feel the over-stuffed feeling. Feel the unpleasant way that your clothes fit. Think about how you physically feel and then think back on the meal and decide when you should have stopped. Make a mental note of these feelings and recall them the next time you are about to over-eat. Also, when you have avoided over-eating, especially if you were tempted by a favorite meal, dwell on the pleasant effects that result from controlling the temptation. Reinforce the feeling. Congratulate yourself.

Eating slowly is particularly important when eating out. You will have less opportunity to control the portions or content of your food, but you can control how much you ingest. Concentrate on slowing down this week, and make the most of each bite of your food.

# WEEK 15: DARE YOU DINE OUT?

T he great majority of restaurants have absolutely no concern for your health or your weight. On the contrary, their goal is to satisfy your taste buds with high-calorie, huge servings. Most people would be appalled at the fat and calorie content of restaurant dishes. You probably have favorite dishes at certain restaurants and you don't have to completely eliminate that pleasure from your diet, but you should make some

> *When having a smackerel of something with a friend, don't eat so much that you get stuck in the doorway trying to get out.*
> *- Pooh's Little Instruction Book, inspired by A. A. Milne*

changes in your choices. Concentrate this week on how to manage caloric intake from restaurants. Here are a few suggestions to help:

**Before leaving for the restaurant:**

- Choose a restaurant that offers many options and that is geared towards healthy eating. There are new health conscious eateries opening everywhere. Be adventurous and try one.

- Have a light (100 calorie) snack such as a bowl of soup, crackers or a cup of tea about thirty minutes before leaving for the restaurant.

- Decide what you are going to eat *before* you go. Almost every restaurant will have healthy, low-calorie options. Remember how good you will feel after the meal by avoiding that bloated feeling and loss of control. Visualize this. By the time you get to the restaurant, your mind will be set and your taste will anticipate the healthier choice.

- *Write in your food journal what you are going to eat.* If you don't know exactly what is on the menu, generalize. If you're going to a seafood restaurant, *plan* to eat a grilled entree with rice rather than fried entree with french fries. This will give you incentive to make better choices when they are placed in front of you on a menu.

**Deciding what to order:**

- Read the menu and deliberately look for the healthy choices while avoiding the unhealthy ones. Don't even read the others. Avoid ingredients such as cheese, cream sauces, bacon, mayonnaise, avocados, nuts, sour cream, and butter. Pile on the mustard, salsa, mushrooms, lettuce, tomatoes, onions and pickles.

- Opt for broiled, grilled, poached or baked items rather then fried or sauteed.

- Whenever possible, ask for sauces or dressings on the side. You should be the one to determine how much of a dressing to use. Dip your fork into the dressing first, then spear your pasta or lettuce. Use the dressing as a condiment rather than a sauce.

- Avoid buffets and "all you can eat" options. Or, start with a salad and make a second trip, fifteen minutes later, for the entree.

- Order a la carte. The "value meal" or the "special" are usually specially priced but have over-sized portions. Remember that eating healthy is often less expensive than eating unwisely. You can afford to spend a bit more while eating out to get exactly what you want—a meal that is healthy and satisfying. You'll make up for the extra money on the days that you don't eat out.

- Order an appetizer or child's meal as your main course. Be cautious, however, because many children's meals consist of nothing but fried items.

- Split a main course with someone.

- Consider ordering soup as an appetizer (not a cream based soup, but a broth or vegetable based.)

- Don't hesitate to ask the server about their healthier choices, serving a smaller portion, or preparing the food in a different way, such as baking rather than frying. Any good restaurant manager will listen to their customers and provide what they want. Many restaurants also have Nutrition Facts on some of their entrees, especially those with claims of healthy content.

- When ordering a side dish, avoid french fries, baked potato with sour cream and butter, potato salad, mayonnaise based cole slaw, and pasta salads with oil based dressings. Opt for steamed vegetables, potato with salsa, vinegar based cole slaw, fresh bread or broth based soups. Avoid vegetables that are stewed in margarine or butter.

- Ask the server to bring you only half of the usual serving. You may have to pay the same price, but it will be much easier for you to stick with a reasonable serving if that is all that is put before you.

- If you order a full sized entree, decide beforehand to eat only half and take half home. This way you get to enjoy your favorite dish twice.

- Most restaurant desserts are large enough for two or three servings. If you can't avoid the dessert list altogether, agree to share one with someone at your table. Opt for items such as key-lime pie, frozen yogurt, angel food cake, berries and powdered sugar. Avoid pies, chocolate and cream based items. If you do order pie, avoid eating the crust which often contains most of the fat.

**Appetizers and waiting for your meal:**

Many restaurants serve chips or bread before the meal is served. You can easily load up on calories and fat from these appetizers long before your meal comes. Here are a few tips to keep this under control:

- Chew gum until your meal is served.

- Put a reasonable portion of chips on a napkin. Limit yourself to this.

- Ask the waiter to remove the appetizer.

- Bring your own appetizer of cut raw vegetables, or toasted pita chips.

- If bread is served, avoid butter and spreads.

**While Eating:**

- *Eat slowly.* This is so important. Give your body time to register fullness before you overeat.

- If your food is not cooked as you expected, or contains much more fat than you anticipated, send it back. The restaurant needs to know what customers want. The food probably is too high in fat if you feel a coating on your teeth, or if your lips feel slippery.

- Be careful at the salad bar. Most salad bars have pastas, tacos, cheese sauces, creamy dressings, fried croutons, nuts, mayonnaise based potato salad or cole slaw, chicken wings, and many other items that are have turned the traditional salad bar into a high-fat smorgasbord. Try a low-fat dressing or mix half low-fat and half regular dressing. If you have a favorite low-calorie dressing at home, bring it along. Leave off the cheese, olives, bacon bits, etc. Fill up on greens. You may be better off opting for a hot bowl of vegetable soup.

Use this week to examine what it is about a certain restaurant that triggers you to overeat. Perhaps you are not overeating every time, but rather, you are eating out too often. If you cannot reduce the calorie content or the portions of what you eat at a restaurant, then you must reduce the *number of times* you eat there. Eating at your favorite restaurant once a month will not ruin your weight control plan. Eating there once or twice a week is how you build fat and lose control. Do you have several restaurants that are a problem? If so, tackle one this week, and write in your food journal, about six weeks from now to tackle another. Get them under control one by one. Then you can enjoy those meals without the guilt.

# WEEK 16: PRODUCE THE PRODUCE

Yes, of course you hate fruits and vegetables! If you loved them, you probably would not be overweight. There are not many vegetarians who are overweight. That is because you can almost eat as many fruits and vegetables as you want without gaining weight. The more you eat, the less likely you are to eat other more fattening foods.

I realize that it's fruitless just to say "eat more produce." If your palate is used to highly refined concentrated sugars and fatty foods, you will not be satisfied with a piece of fruit. As in all the steps we have taken so far, we will sneak this in gradually and without pain. You will develop a taste for fruits and veggies and replace those cravings for high-calorie foods with cravings for nutritious food.

> *I do not like broccoli. And I haven't liked it since I was a little kid and my mother made me eat it. And I'm President of the United States and I'm not going to eat any more broccoli.*
> *- President George Bush, 1990*

The variety of fresh produce in this country is astounding. And most fruits and vegetables are available, fresh or frozen, all year long. Use this week to add one vegetable or fruit serving every day. So if you now eat only two portions of vegetables a day, eat three. Check your journal entries and see how many portions of fruits and vegetables you are eating. I bet you'll be shocked. None, one, maybe two portions a day? The recommended is *three to five portions of vegetables and two to three servings of fruits per day.* Add this serving without adding calories to your day. **Your goal is to *replace* about 100 calories of a less nutritional choice with a fruit or vegetable serving.** For instance, rather than the midday soft drink, have an apple.

Note that this means unprocessed fruits and vegetables. Avoid canned fruits because they are usually canned in heavy syrup. They have also lost many of their vitamins and nutrients. Canned vegetables usually have added salt or sugar. Frozen vegetables and fruits are fine if they do not have added sauces, sugars or salt. Dried fruits are great for traveling or the lunchbox, but some can be high in calories and contain sulfites. Remember, the foods to look for are those that are the least processed. Picked from your own garden would be the best.

Look at different varieties and try something you have never had before. How about a rutabaga? Papaya? Kale? Yellow-eyed peas? Kiwi fruit? Be brave! Don't get discouraged. Keep trying until you find some great new choices. And try each variety more than once. You may have gotten a piece of fruit that wasn't quite ripe or just not the pick of the crop. Some will be better than others. Ask the produce manager how to pick the best of a certain variety of produce. The difference between a good cantaloupe and a bad one is enormous. And this is usually true of most produce.

Spend time in the library or bookstore exploring recipes for vegetables. Look for recipes that will allow you to incorporate new fruits and vegetables in your menus.

Give yourself the best possible chance to like produce by buying the best. Buy the freshest and don't avoid the most expensive. Your food bill is going to be much less while eating healthy so you can afford to buy the best produce. A two dollar fresh pineapple may be just OK, but the four dollar pineapple from Hawaii might be outstanding. And you will remember that taste next time you want something sweet.

For the best tasting and freshest produce, buy what is in season and what is grown locally. Often the best produce will be at a corner produce stand rather than the national food chain. Avoid buying enough fresh vegetables for the whole week. If you can't get to the market every day, only get fresh vegetables for the first couple days. Then rely on frozen for the rest of the week.

If you worry about the effect of residual pesticides in produce, research indicates that the nutritional benefits of increased produce in your diet far outweighs the risks that exist from residual pesticides. You can reduce your risk of ingesting pesticides by buying domestic produce. Imported produce is more likely to be contaminated than U.S. produce (with the exception of U.S. cherries which often test higher in residual pesticides than imported cherries.) You can also reduce the levels of pesticides by thoroughly washing. In general, fruits will have higher levels of pesticides (strawberries are by far the most contaminated) than vegetables. Fruits have a higher sugar content than vegetables, and therefore are more attractive to pests, so more pesticides are used to increase the harvest.

You can, of course, buy organic products which should be free from pesticides. Pesticides are the price we pay for unblemished, lower cost, pest free food. Personally, I would prefer to see a worm on my ear of corn than to wonder if the bitter taste was a big mouthful of poison. If it's good enough for that worm, it's probably good enough for me.

# WEEK 17: WHAT'S YOUR PLEASURE?

W hat's this? How does this relate to weight management? Actually, you are about to build a powerful list of items that can help you through those moments of weakness. In the past, you may have overeaten as reward, celebration, to reduce stress, or for comfort. Whatever the reason, you used food to gain pleasure or reduce discomfort. This week, concentrate on other things that give you those same feelings.

Food is for fuel and sustenance. Yes, eating will always be pleasurable, but when overeating results in an unhealthy and unhappy lifestyle, the momentary

**Turn your appetite for food into an appetite for fun.**

pleasure is too high a price to pay. Indulge in those pleasures that do not come with unhealthy side effects.

You will have times when your resolve is low. Everyone does. When those times occur, rather than reaching for a bag of chips, grab your list of fun things instead. As you do this you will be conditioning yourself to do your favorite things for reward, pleasure or comfort rather than eating. Each time will be easier and easier until it is finally second nature. You will not only have fun and pleasure, but also the long lasting knowledge that you have made a better choice makes you stronger each time.

Use this week to reach back into your experiences and list those things that you find fun. Use the chart at the end of the chapter. Here are some examples:

- Play board games or cards with your children or grandchildren.

- Get a bird feeder.

- Take your kids to a community play.

- Pick up a new hobby such as needlework, woodworking, whittling, carving, painting, or photography.

- Plan a white water rafting trip.

- Learn to play an instrument.

- Learn flyfishing.

- Join your kids for lunch at their school.

- Take a trip to a nearby city and see the sites.

- Take a drive in the country. During the day enjoy the countryside, and stargaze at night.

- Go to a movie, or rent one. Get a great comedy.

- Have sex.

- Take a hot bubble bath.

- Get a facial or massage.

- Write. Keep a journal or write a letter to a long lost friend or elderly relative.

- Read. Go to the library and browse.

- Put on the headphones and listen to a CD.

- Sign up for scuba diving lessons.

- Go skydiving.

- Learn how to juggle.

- Get a directory of classes from a local community college and sign up. Learn more about investing, crafts, parenting or gardening.

Reach outside of your own experiences and list things that you've never done, yet want to. How about some pleasures that you used to enjoy when you were younger and/or thinner? The next time you reach for food for any reason other than fuel, reach for your list. Try it this week. Have fun and congratulate yourself.

## List of Fun Things

# WEEK 18: BEVERAGE LEVERAGE

Igh calorie drinks (colas, lemonade, alcohol, whole milk, sweetened ice tea, juices, etc.) usually account for many calories in an over-eater's diet. Juices and skim milk are nutritious but must be considered as a serving from the fruit or milk group. Sugared drinks and alcohol, on the other hand, add nothing but empty calories to your diet. If you already have control of high-calorie drinks in your diet, use this week to reinforce the habits from the previous weeks, or move on to the next week. If you love your sugared drinks, don't panic. This will be easy. By now you should be drinking 64 ounces of water each day and this has probably lessened your craving for other drinks, including those with alcohol or sugar. Many people can easily lose ten to twenty pounds in a year simply by eliminating colas. Just one, twelve ounce cola has 155 calories, which is equivalent to nine teaspoons of sugar. *One per day for a year equals sixteen pounds.*

As mentioned earlier, I do not strictly adhere to each and every tip in this book. I use some occasionally, some often, and some religiously. This is one that I practice without exception. I prefer not to drink my calories. I have not had a sugared drink in probably fifteen years and don't miss it a bit. Occasionally I will sip

Don't Diet—*Live It!*

sugared tea or cola by mistake, and the taste is rather sickeningly, syrupy sweet.

You don't have to eliminate sugared drinks altogether this week. If this has been a regular element of your diet for years that would be an unlikely request. Modify your intake every day so that by the end of the year you have met your goal. To do this, try one of these methods:

- Cut each serving in half. If you normally have a twelve ounce soft drink, have six ounces instead. Buy the drink in plastic bottles that you can put the top on, and save the other half for the next time you would normally have a soda. Pour it in a glass with ice. This will give you the sense of a large serving.

- Reduce the number of times per day that you have a sugared drink. If you regularly have two glasses of sweetened tea with lunch, change that to one glass of tea and one glass of water.

- Mix your drink half and half with the diet variety. For sodas, you can mix half diet with half regular soda. For iced tea, you can use half sugar and half non-sugar sweetener to your drink. Better yet, lower the amount of total sweetening that you use. Your palate will gradually adjust to and actually prefer the sweet taste in lower and lower concentrations.

- Replace the sugared drink with another drink such as unsweetened tea, sparkling water, or optimally, just plain water. Sparkling water with a splash of orange juice makes a great drink.

An added benefit to reducing sweetened drinks is that you will probably be eliminating a great deal of caffeine also. Most colas and teas have caffeine which compounds stress and upsets your sleeping patterns, which will make your goals harder to achieve. Caffeine late in the day or evening can also cause nightmares or disturbing dreams. Be aware that if you try to eliminate all caffeine immediately, you can suffer severe headaches. The way to avoid this is to eliminate the caffeine drinks gradually, as suggested here. In addition to reducing caffeine and calories, you'll also undoubtedly save a good bit of money. One fifty cent cola a day adds up to $182 in a year. You could use that $182 to do some of the Fun Things that you listed last week.

Keeping yourself hydrated will help you immensely in this effort. Hopefully you have developed a habit of drinking at least 64 ounces of water each day. (If not, you should revisit Week 8: The Water Way.) Next time you are tempted to grab a soda or beer, tell yourself you'll have it after you drink twelve ounces of water. You probably will forget all about the soda after you've quenched your thirst.

Drop your intake one quarter this week, by one of the methods above. In your food journal two months from now, make a note to cut back another quarter. Do this again two months from that, and then finally eliminate sweetened drinks all together. Be sure to keep an eye on your total intake of calorie and insure that you are not replacing those calories with extra food.

# WEEK 19: TOO MUCH OF A GOOD THING

Y ou may be eating all the right foods but if your portions are out of control, you will never gain control of your weight. The great thing about portion control is that it allows you to eat all your favorite foods. It's all about moderation. Let's look at some ways to gain control of portions:

- Get a small kitchen scale, and for this week, *weigh or measure everything you eat.* Guess what it weighs before weighing. When you are very good at estimation you can use the scale periodically just to be sure. Weigh out a three ounce piece of chicken and take a good look at it. How much space does it take up on the plate? Is it about the size of your palm? How thick is it? A half-inch thick piece of meat does not look much bigger than a quarter-inch piece but has twice the fat and calories.

- It is especially important to monitor your portions of meats and fats because the calorie content of these foods is so concentrated and high relative to fruits, vegetables and starches. An oversized serving of vegetables is not nearly as damaging as an oversized serving of meat, french fries or a couple extra tablespoons of ranch salad dressing.

- Measure your carbohydrates also. Though not as damaging as meats and fats, starches can add considerably to your total daily caloric intake. Carbohydrates from refined, processed grains, such as white flour and white rice, should be more carefully measured than those from whole grains.

- You can be less accurate with fruits, and even less accurate with vegetables. It won't matter nearly as much if you have twice the vegetable serving, in fact, it will probably benefit you.

- Most salad dressings are extremely high in fat and are measured in terms of one tablespoon. Measure out a tablespoon and see how it covers your salad. You may be surprised to discover that you are actually lopping on a half cup and 80 grams of fat on your salad, while thinking you are eating light. You can easily ingest as many fat calories from salad dressing as are in a full blown double cheeseburger and french fry meal. Get a pump bottle, such as a hand soap pump, for your thicker dressings. You will do much better by pumping it on your salad rather than spooning or pouring from a wide-mouthed bottle. Measure how many pumps it takes to fill a tablespoon. You can put thinner dressings, such as oil, vinegar or lemon in a spray bottle which will give great coverage and avoid pooling in the bottom of the bowl. Another way to control the amount of dressing you use it to always get it on the side. Dip your fork into the dressing (or sauce or gravy), then spear your food.

- Measure out a tablespoon of mayonnaise or butter and see how it spreads on a piece of bread. Find out exactly how much butter you use on your morning toast, or how much mayonnaise you use in a sandwich.

- Measure the cooking oil that you use to stir fry. Pour one tablespoon into the pan and move it around with a spatula or paper towel to coat the entire surface. You don't need five to six tablespoons to stir fry. In fact, a coating of cooking spray is all you need. If you have a non-stick pan, you won't even need the cooking spray.

- If you eat ice cream or frozen yogurt, scoop out one-half cup, then put it into your usual bowl to see what the volume looks like.

- A good way to control portions is to cook or serve food in serving-sized dishes. For instance, rather than baking a layered cake, bake cupcakes. You can also bake 30 cupcakes rather than 24, using the same amount of batter. Bake your turkey stuffing (dressing) in muffin pans, and serve as a "stuffin". Look for the small bowls that cafeterias use for portion control—sometimes called "monkey dishes". Rather than heaping an undeterminable amount of potatoes or pasta onto your dinner plate, use these smaller side dishes.

- Pay attention to the Serving Size and number of servings per package on the Nutrition Facts Labels. If the item says "three servings per package" then be sure that you divide that up into three equal portions. You will often find out that a

> *All the things I really like to do are either immoral, illegal, or fattening.*
> *- Alexander Woollcott*

package that looks like a single serving is actually two or three servings. If you eat the entire package, you'll have to multiply the calories by the number of servings.

As you become more adept at judging portion sizes at home, you will judge portions at restaurants more accurately. You will find that most servings at restaurants are far larger than the USDA definition for a "serving." In fact, usually the appetizers alone in a restaurant are more than a full sized serving. Desserts can be easily equivalent to three or four servings. The only thing restaurants seem to skimp on is fruit and vegetable servings. The typical restaurant adult entree rarely exemplifies the recommendations in the Food Guide Pyramid. The following chart illustrates examples of serving sizes.

# The Pyramid Guide to Daily Food Choices

| Food Group | Per day | Examples of one serving |
|---|---|---|
| Breads, Cereals, Rice, Pastas<br>Choose whole grains, and watch out for added sugar, salt and fat. | 6 – 11 | 1 slice bread<br>½ burger bun or English muffin<br>6 small crackers<br>½ cup cooked cereal<br>¾ – 1 cup dry cereal<br>½ cup rice or pasta |
| Vegetables<br>Choose fresh or frozen vegetables. Avoid sauces. | 3 – 5 | ½ cup cooked or chopped raw vegetables<br>1 cup leafy raw vegetable |
| Fruits<br>Choose fresh fruit, or canned in it's own juice. Avoid fruit canned in heavy syrup. | 2 – 3 | 1 whole medium fruit<br>½ larger fruit<br>½ cup fresh berries<br>½ cup canned fruit<br>½ cup juice |
| Milk, cheese and yogurt<br>Choose low-fat items. Avoid yogurts with added sugar. | 2 – 4 | 1 cup milk<br>8 oz or 1 cup yogurt<br>1–2 ounces cheese |
| Meat, fish, poultry, dry beans, eggs and nuts<br>Choose low-fat items. | 2 – 3 | 2–3 ounces lean meat, fish or poultry<br>1 egg<br>½ cup cooked dry beans<br>2 Tblsp seeds or nuts |
| Oils and fats<br>Use sparingly; calories from fat should not exceed 30% of daily calories | | 1 tsp oil or butter<br>1 tblsp prepared oil based dressing |

Note: The guide to daily food choices described here was developed for Americans who regularly eat foods from all the major food groups listed. Some people such as vegetarians and others may not eat one or more of these types of foods. These people may wish to contact a dietitian or nutritionist for help in planning food choices.

Source: Using The Food Guide Pyramid: A Resource for Nutrition Educators U.S. Department of Agriculture Food, Nutrition, and Consumer Services Center For Nutrition Policy and Promotion, 1995

Check yourself often through the weeks ahead to insure that your portions are not creeping up. An extra 100 calories a day can add up to ten pounds a year. You may be eating exactly the same *things* as someone who has their weight under control and wonder why you are not losing weight. The difference is probably that the other person is eating controlled portions—starting with less, refusing seconds and even leaving some uneaten.

# WEEK 20: WANNA DANCE?

Last quarter, you altered your everyday movements to increase your activity. This week, you will choose an activity that you can look forward to and that has benefits in addition to losing weight.

Exercising for the sheer sake of losing weight is a terrific waste of human energy. Ever wonder where the world would be if we could focus the energy of all the "exercisers" in this country towards actual goals? Fat tissue is nothing but stored energy. Burned fat = work. Why waste that energy? That is like leaving your car running until it is out of gas. You can exercise like a hamster in a treadmill, or you can actually achieve end results (in addition to losing weight, toning and improving health) with your excess fuel.

> *The only reason I would take up jogging is so I could hear heavy breathing again.*
> *-Erma Bombeck*

In addition to adding small increases in daily activity as mentioned in the first quarter, choose a life enriching activity that has benefits far greater (but including) weight loss and health maintenance. This can be a hobby, a sport, or a volunteer activity. Some examples are:

- Get involved in your child's sport or sponsor a foster child in a sport such as soccer. Take them to practice and games, and help with practices. Practice with the child at home on regular, predetermined times. Be a coach or assistant coach for a youth or adult team such as baseball. Call your local YMCA for information.

- Walk briskly in your neighborhood with your support partner, your child, your pet or a neighbor. Have a great conversation. If you are like many of folks who cannot exercise outdoors because of allergies, visit an indoor mall and walk there. Many malls open before the individual stores just for walkers. It's safe, climate controlled, no inclines or car fumes, and you can window shop while you walk.

- Take dancing lessons with your spouse. Rekindle the relationship.

- Take a local elementary school class on a trip in a nearby park.

- Teach your dog how to catch a ball or Frisbee. Not only will you improve his quality of life, but also his general behavior. Volunteer at your local Humane Society Shelter and walk the dogs that are crying for attention.

Choose an activity or two that interests you and commit to spending at least sixty minutes, cumulatively, each week. Ideally, you want to break this sixty minutes among three days. For instance, walk for twenty minutes each on Monday, Wednesday and Friday. Try not to be too rigid in your scheduling, however. Be flexible, but make sure you get in at least sixty minutes of activity by the end of the week. Ease yourself into increased activity, just as you ease yourself into the Food Guide Pyramid model. By the end of the year, you will *enjoy* your increased energy and activity level.

Choosing an activity that is rewarding and fun is an important way to insure that you get the exercise you need. Here are some other tips to insure your success:

> *Life is short; live it up.*
> *-Nikita Krushchev*

- Get the proper equipment, especially shoes and clothing. Go to a sports store and try on several pairs of shoes. I've had shoes that felt so good that I actually *wanted* to put them on and run. In week 23, you'll see how much money you'll save while losing weight, and this is an excellent way to spend those savings.

- Use music as a tool to help you maintain rhythm and interest. You can also use music as a timing device. Make a tape of several of your favorite songs that amount to twenty minutes.

- Get information on the sport, hobby or topic. Rent a video, find books or subscribe to a related magazine. A periodical that comes to your mailbox once a month is a great motivator and reminder to stick with it. Get involved in a local chapter of a group devoted to the activity. Learn about the best equipment for your sport, the best locations, and safety tips. By learning and participating, you are developing the mindset of a fit person.

- Record your activity for the coming week in your food journal. Plan for it. This is particularly important during the holidays or while on a vacation when our schedules are harried and different.

- Schedule your activity at a convenient and available time. The best time would be that time of day that you typically over-eat.

- If the weather doesn't cooperate, have a backup plan. This is where a stationary bike or treadmill will come in handy. I would not recommend this for a regular activity because it can become quite boring. However, when it's been raining for days, or you simply can't get out of the house, a thirty minute session can be stress-relieving. You can read, watch television, listen to a book-on-tape or music to pass the time.

In coming weeks, we will increase this activity until, at the end of the year, you are exercising thirty minutes on most days of the week.

Don't Diet—*Live It!*

# WEEK 21: GET OUT OF THAT RUT

T his entire year is about change. You are slowly but deliberately making monumental changes in your lifestyle. You have acknowledged that your lifestyle needs change. Change, even if positive, is sometimes difficult to deal with and accept. But change can be exciting, rewarding and a sign of growth.

We often get stuck in a rut that reminds us of our past habits and hinders the growth of new habits. For instance, let's say that everyday for the last five years, you've come home, dropped in your favorite chair and enjoyed two beers before dinner. If you continue to come home at the same time, drop into the same chair, watch the same TV program, your body is going to expect those two beers. Resisting that temptation would be quite difficult. If, on the other hand, you came home, took your dog for a walk (who would be ecstatic at this new attention), then you would not be so inclined to follow through on that old ritual.

*You will find that your old routines no longer fit your new role, just as your old clothes no longer fit your new body.*

You are sculpting a new body and a new image. Your body, clothes, skin, ring size, maybe even your shoe size will change. You will smile more. You will be more active and appear younger. Other people will see you differently. This is a new role for you. You will find that your old routines no longer fit your new role, just as your old clothes no longer fit your new body.

This week, look at your routines and make some positive changes. Change is growth. If you find change particularly difficult, it may help to start making small changes in your daily routines and environment. Here are some examples:

- Switch sides of the bed.

- Light candles at dinner.

- Go back to school. Take a community class or start work towards a degree.

- Change your route to work.

- Consider changing your work hours, or even changing jobs.

- Rearrange a room in your house or your office.

- Take all the pictures down in your home, and put new photos or pictures in the frames.

- Plan a weekend getaway today for this weekend.

- Rearrange your refrigerator. Put the healthy things in front at eye level.

- Open the windows.

- Have breakfast for dinner.

- Turn off the TV and read tonight.

- Change your hair.

These small changes may seem insignificant, but they will prepare your mind to accept the more profound changes that will improve your lifestyle.

# WEEK 22: LOTSA PASTA

C urrent guidelines recommend eating six to eleven servings of starches per day. That's six servings for smaller people and eleven for taller, large frame individuals. Starches should make up the bulk of your diet. Not all starches are nutritious however. Here's a breakdown:

*Breads.* Go for bagels, bran muffins (but watch the fat and sugar), English muffin, or a slice of any type of bread, especially breads with whole grains. Avoid croissant rolls, buttered garlic bread, donuts, cakes, breakfast biscuits (usually high in saturated fat), canned biscuits, and croutons.

*Rices.* Choose rice seasoned with broth, spices and vegetables, or plain rice. Powdered butter flavoring is great on steamed rice. Usually rice served in Oriental restaurants is low in fat, with the exception of fried rice. Avoid minute rice (low in calories but also low in nutrients), packaged rice mixes (high in salt, sugar, MSG), fried rice and Mexican rice in restaurants. Rice makes a perfect bed for stir fried dishes, or a base for burritos and fajitas. It's a great staple to keep in the pantry.

***Pastas.*** Pasta by itself is a great addition to a healthy diet. It's the sauces that are usually a problem. Opt for tomato or vegetable based sauces. When making cold pasta salads, use equal amounts of vegetables to pasta. Go easy on the olives. Drizzle the dressing on just before serving. If you put the dressing on hours before serving, the pasta will absorb it, and you will need more to taste it. If you really need cheese in your pasta, sprinkle some on top rather than mixing throughout the dish. Avoid pasta made with eggs, pasta mixes, and cream or cheese based sauces.

Many pasta dishes use a relatively small amount of pasta. Stuffed pastas such as manicotti and ravioli tend to be high in calories because they are stuffed with cheese and meat. Lasagna can be extremely high in calories, but you can also find (and make) relatively healthy lasagnas. A sausage lasagna laden with olive oil, ricotta from whole milk and provolone can easily have many times the calories of a lasagna made with spinach, fat-free tomato sauce, low-fat ricotta and mozzarella.

Try different varieties of pasta, such as tomato, spinach, and whole wheat. Try different brands. Experiment making your own pasta, or buying it fresh. Fresh pasta will have a very different taste than dried.

***Cereals.*** Dried cereals can make a great light snack. Choose Shredded Wheat, Puffed Wheat, Grape Nuts, Corn Flakes, Chex, Rice Crispies, Cheerios or other low-sugar cereals. Splash on skim milk and add a few slices of banana, peach, or berries and you've got a near perfect breakfast. Avoid granolas which are usually high in calories and fat, and of course sugar cereals. These would be a better fit for the cookie and candy aisle.

*Crackers.* Choose low-sodium soup crackers, or Melba toast. Read the labels carefully on the crackers you choose. The majority have high-sodium and fat content. Make your own pita chips: cut pita bread into triangles and toast, with or without seasonings. Try different types of pita breads: whole wheat, sesame seed, etc.

*Potatoes.* Potatoes are the mainstay of many American diets. Without adornment, a potato is a great starch to add to your regular diet. Avoid french fries, fattening toppings on a baked potato, too much butter in whipped potatoes and heavy cream sauce. Experiment with toppings such as salsa, non-fat sour cream, plain yogurt, chives, garlic, basil and nutmeg. You can easily make a baked potato a nutritious meal. Be sure to eat the skin as well. A terrific substitute for french fries is baked fries: french cut potatoes or slice thin. Peeling is optional. Mix a couple of egg whites with your favorite seasoned salt. Dip the potatoes in the egg mixture. Bake at 400 degrees, turning every 15 minutes, for a total of 45 minutes.

This week, examine the balance of starches in your food journal. Too much or too little? Aim for the recommended six to eleven servings. Remember that a serving is one slice of bread, one half English muffin, six small crackers, one half cup cooked rice or pasta, one half cup cooked cereal, or three quarters to one cup dry cereal. Replace one serving from the meat group with one serving from the starch group each day. Of course, if your diet already consists of six to eleven servings, then look at those choices and see how you can change them into more nutritious choices with the tips above. Concentrate on those starches and move closer to your goal.

# WEEK 23: COUNT YOUR BLESSINGS

W hat a fun week this will be. Use this week to cash in on a great benefit of eating healthy—saving money! Without question, in most countries, eating healthy is less expensive than eating a poor diet. You should be eating less, and eating foods with fewer calories and that are less processed. The foods that are expensive are those that are fast, processed and high in calories.

The most expensive cuts of meat often are highest in fat content. For instance, a rib eye steak is 50% fat, as compared to top round which is 25% fat. The most expensive salmon also contains the highest fat content. For chicken and turkey, however, the most expensive white meat cuts are lower in fat than dark meat.

Dried beans, rice, potatoes, turkey or chicken breast (not processed or deli meat), and water instead of colas, are all healthy and inexpensive substitutions in your diet. If you eliminate buying one soda from a vending machine every work day of the year, at 75 cents each, you can save $150. Eliminating one trip to a fast food restaurant for four dollars every week can save $208. Fat is expensive. Only kings could be fat centuries ago, but today, even our pets are fat.

You will also be saving money in health bills. This will be more difficult to calculate, unless you are already paying a premium on your medical insurance for an obesity related illness. Most of your health benefits will be long term such as a reduced need for medications, increased life expectancy, reduced risk of diabetes, stroke and heart attack, speedier recovery from illness and injury, etc.

You will save money in clothes. As you lose weight you will be able to wear more styles and choose from a larger variety of clothes and stores. Your clothes will not wear out as fast due to stressed seams.

Calculate your savings and each week put this away in a separate jar or bank account. Use this money to celebrate your great success at established milestones, for instance for every ten pounds lost, or the end of the each quarter.

# WEEK 24: GET THE LARD OUT

A major portion of your fat intake is probably from meats. Fat from meat—lard or saturated fat—is the most dangerous type of fat. There are many ways you can continue to eat meat but reduce the intake of fat. You don't have to become a vegetarian. We will devote this week and another week in the fourth quarter to examining this issue. To get started, try a few of these tips:

*Oppose adipose to close your clothes.*

- You can dramatically reduce fat from ground meats with a few simple tricks. Ground beef and ground sausage can be quite high in fat. Start with meat that has the lowest fat content. Cook it completely, until it is well browned. Drain off all the fat that you can. Then either roll and press the meat between several layers of paper towels, or rinse in a colander with hot water. Even processed this way, ground sausage will still have a good deal of fat so you should use it sparingly. If you grill a hamburger, drain it and press it between several sheets of paper towels before serving.

- Choose leaner cuts of every kind of meat. For poultry and pork, choose white meat. For beef, choose eye of the round and top round. Unfortunately, the most tender cuts also have the most fat. To tenderize leaner cuts, use a marinade, meat tenderizer, or a meat pounder.

- Always trim all visible fat off of meat before cooking. The fat on poultry will be just under the skin, so remove the skin as well.

- Cook all meats until they are well-done. Meat that is cooked rare will retain much more fat than meat cooked well-done. As the temperature of the meat rises, more and more fat melts away. Cooking thoroughly will also reduce the level of bacteria and parasites that might be present in meat.

- Cook your meats in such a way that the fat can drain. For instance, place your roast on a slotted tray or rack inside the roasting pan. Cook your hamburgers, chops or steaks on the grill rather than in a fry pan.

- Use an extender in your ground meats such as cooked lentils or other legumes, or crushed cereal like shredded wheat, Chex or corn flakes, oatmeal, texturized vegetable protein (TVP) or crushed saltine crackers. Use one part extender to two parts ground meat.

- Substitute Canadian bacon for regular bacon or pepperoni. Regular bacon is extremely high in fat and sodium and should be avoided. Canadian bacon, on the other hand is very lean and makes and excellent meat for breakfast, in a biscuit sandwich, crumbled on a salad or on a BLT (bacon lettuce tomato) sandwich. Canadian bacon is also a great substitute for pepperoni on pizzas. As an example, an English muffin with two slices of Canadian bacon has 170 calories and 3 grams of fat, as compared to a fast food bacon biscuit which has 420 calories and 28 grams of fat. If you must occasionally have bacon, discard all the lard which melts off during cooking. Don't be tempted to use this to cook other items.

- Avoid packaged meats such as bologna, hot-dogs, sausages, etc. Not only are they laden with excess fat and sodium, they also contain preservatives and additives. They are also made of the least desirable cuts of meat.

- Buy canned tuna packed in water (two ounces is 60 calories and 2 grams of fat) instead of packed in oil (two ounces is 100 calories and 8 grams of fat.)

- Choose fish, turkey and chicken breast more often than red meat. When choosing pork, try lean chops or a lean roast rather than bacon or sausage. Gradually reduce the number of meals you have with red meat. Replace with vegetarian, fish or fowl entrees.

- Avoid deli meats and luncheon meats. Most are highly processed and have added sugar, preservatives, salt and fat. They are more expensive and they certainly do not taste as good as the real thing. Look carefully at a package of lunch meat. If you calculate the per pound price, it will often be three times higher than buying fresh meat.

# WEEK 25: GO LOW SODIUM

**M**ost American diets are much too high in sodium, or salt. Sodium is essential for muscle contraction and hydration, however, too much sodium can cause serious medical conditions such as high blood pressure, and can result in excess water retention. One of the reasons our diets are so high in sodium is that most prepackaged foods have high amounts of added sodium. You will see quick results in weight loss when you reduce your intake of salt. This will be strictly water weight, but can give you added motivation to stick to your goals.

The amount of salt that you need in your food to achieve a certain "taste" depends on what your palate is used to. As you gradually reduce the amount of salt you consume, your palate will adjust to the point where salty foods are very unpleasant. If you currently can eat a serving of regular packaged potato chips, then you are ingesting too much sodium. After you've adjusted to lower sodium levels, those potato chips will be almost impossible for you to eat. Most processed foods are unnecessarily high in sodium. As you reduce your taste for sodium, you will reduce your taste for most processed foods which are also high in calories and fat. Look at the Nutrition Facts labels for sodium content. Items that are typically high in added salt are:

- Soups, even those advertising 30% less sodium, will often still be too high.
- Tomato based vegetable juices—just for an experiment, buy the sodium free variety. You will be shocked at how much salt you must add to equal the taste of the regular variety.
- Frozen entrees, even diet varieties. These might be low-calorie or low-fat, but may be very high in sodium.
- Packaged rice or pasta mixes. Any mix that includes a "spice sack."
- Deli meats
- Dry breakfast cereals
- Potato chips and other snack chips
- Salsas and dips
- Cheeses
- Many pickled foods
- Soy sauce
- Spices or processed foods that contain monosodium glutamate (MSG)

Tips to reduce sodium:

- Move towards eliminating table salt. Buy salt shakers with smaller holes. This really works.

- Taste your food before salting it. This might sound obvious, but many people habitually salt their food even before they've sampled it.

- Most foods in their unprocessed state are naturally low in sodium. Avoid processed foods as much as possible.

- Limit the times that you dine out. Restaurant meals (especially fast food) usually contain excess fat, calories, portions and sodium.

- If you want to try a salt substitute, be sure to check with your health care provider. Some salt substitutes can interfere with the absorption of some medications.

- Avoid adding salt during cooking. Let each person decide for themselves how much salt to use. Your taste for salt can be dramatically different from theirs. Also, you can use less salt and get the same taste if it's sprinkled on top just before eating rather than mixed throughout the dish.

- Leave salt out of cold salads such as potato salad or cole slaw. Adding salt will draw water out of the potatoes, making the salad watery as it chills.

- Use pepper, spices, lemon, vinegars or wine to flavor your foods.

- If you buy canned vegetables or beans that contain sodium, rinse before using. Most canned goods contain added salt, and sometimes added sugars.

- If you bite into an item that tastes too salty, stop eating it. Eating overly salted foods will train your palate to crave more.

- Try some of the lower sodium packaged foods. Sometimes the sodium-free varieties are not palatable, but the reduced sodium versions can be quite good.

# Week 26: Second Quarter Review

This is the half way mark! Congratulations! If you have persisted and taken each week seriously, you are well on your way to changing those old habits *forever*. Your framework for a healthy lifestyle is in place.

Set aside some time each day this week to review each week from the first and second quarter. Look seriously at the task for each week, and decide which ones need work. Write reminders in your food journal in the coming weeks to reinforce the tasks from the last two quarters.

It is time to review your goals. Should they be revised? Are you on track? Are you losing weight too quickly?

Compare your food journal for last week to the first couple of weeks. Where were your greatest successes? Your weaknesses? Your diet should be quite different than it was 26 weeks ago. Review the Week 7: Get the Skinny and see what additional changes you can make in your diet to move closer to the Food Guide Pyramid model.

Pay particular attention to the foundation building tasks in the first few weeks such as keeping a food journal and planning your diet. Both of these should be second nature by now.

Are you impatient to lose weight more quickly? Remind yourself that numerous studies have shown that slow weight loss is much more likely to be permanent weight loss. Perhaps you grew up in a family that reinforced poor eating habits. Use this year as a retraining year and conditioning year. An expert does not become an expert overnight. Just as becoming a star tennis player takes practice, so does becoming thin, in body and mind. Also remember that weight loss is only one objective in this plan—the other more important objective is to live a healthy lifestyle that *results* in a healthy weight.

> *Success seems to be more a matter of hanging on after others have let go.*
> *– William Feather*

Let's review the last quarter and try to reinforce each week with a new idea:

**Make It Last:** Put a clock with a second hand in the room where you eat the most.

**Dare You Dine Out?:** Discard any takeout menus in your home that offer only high-calorie meals.

**Produce the Produce:** Try a kiwi fruit, pared and sliced with your cereal.

**What's Your Pleasure?:** Schedule a favorite activity right now, for a time in the next few days when you are likely to overeat.

**Beverage Leverage:** Be sure that the "fruit" juice you are drinking is 100% fruit juice. *Many* juices are 10% juice with added fructose (sugar). And beware that fruit juice counts as a serving of fruit—watch the calories. An extra eight ounces of juice each day for a year can add up to ten pounds.

*Too Much of a Good Thing:* Measure eight ounces of juice into a drinking glass. Draw a line with a marker at the eight ounce level.

*Wanna Dance?:* Ask a friend, spouse or your kids to come up with some activities that you can do together. They'll have dozens.

*Get Out of That Rut:* Go barefoot.

*Lotsa Pasta:* Find a good neighborhood bakery and try one of their whole grain breads or fresh pastas.

*Count Your Blessings:* Put your savings, dollars and change, into a big clear glass jar and keep it in a visible spot such as on the counter next to the refrigerator. This will be one more reminder of your goal and your progress.

*Get The Lard Out:* Choices of ground beef from leanest to highest fat content are: sirloin, ground round, ground chuck and regular ground beef.

*Go Low Sodium:* Use garlic powder instead of garlic salt. Use salt-free butter (which is usually preferred in recipes.)

# THIRD QUARTER: BRICK LAYING

# WEEK 27: LET'S DO LUNCH

L ast quarter you took control of the breakfast hour. (As with every week of the *Live It!* Plan, if you have not mastered the task of the week, start that week over. Each task builds on the ones before and must all be mastered for success.) This week, we will see how we can modify lunch to move you closer to your weight loss and health goal.

Going out to lunch can be a significant problem for people who are trying to control their weight. Fast food establishments make it painfully easy to overeat, and there is often a

*It's like the coming of civilization.*
*- Anonymous Moscow Resident,*
*opening of the first Russian McDon-*
*alds Restaurant, Moscow, 1990*

willing group of lunch partners at the office. If fast food is your issue, you can do several things to control the amount of calories. Order the smallest size of each item. Order a child's meal instead of the big combo meal. Get a salad instead of fries. Get water instead of a soda. Review the tips in week 12, *Dealing with Restaurants.*

Limit your lunch restaurant visits to only once a week. On the other days of the week, have a planned and prepared meal. Bring your lunch to work. Even if you don't work away from home, pack your lunch anyway the night before.

Try to eat lunch about an hour later than usual. You might try eating all meals one hour later. If it is easier for you to avoid eating in the morning hours, then put breakfast off until mid morning, then have lunch at two o'clock. This way you won't be famished when you get home from work.

Exercise before lunch, then you will be much less inclined to overeat.

If lunch is your primary meal, you may find it very difficult to reduce severely. It would be unwise to abruptly change this routine. I've interviewed folks who have started on a diet with the best of intentions.

*Structure your plan for moderating your diet with success in mind.*

They immediately try to tackle the most difficult area or time of day. For instance, they replace their high–fat, fast food lunch with a liquid diet shake. This is a sure bet for failure. They feel deprived, unsatiated, and ultimately guilty when they cannot follow through. A better plan would be to first tackle those times of day and/or meals that are easiest for you to manage. If you are not very hungry at dinner time, then concentrate your reductions then. Accumulate some successes and confidence, and then use that confidence to tackle the meal that is the toughest for you to moderate. This is not to say that you should not modify your lunch patterns at all this week. Rather, if lunch is your favorite and main meal, then plan your modifications gradually, and concentrate on other times of the day that will be easier for you. However, if you often eat a high–calorie lunch even though you are really not hungry, then this would be a great time to eliminate many unrewarding calories. Everyone has unique tastes, appetites and challenges. Structure your plan for moderating your diet with success in mind.

Review your food journal and see how many calories you typically each at lunch. Try to reduce this by one quarter using the methods we have used many times before: reduce the portion, reduce the number of times you go to a particular restaurant, reduce the calorie content, or make a healthier choice. Six months from now, write in your food journal to reduce your lunch calories by another quarter. Of course, if lunch is not your problem area, you may not need to adjust this drastically. On the other hand, if it is the major source of your calories, then you may even want to reduce another quarter nine months from now.

# WEEK 28: GOOD THINGS ARE GREEN

G reen...and yellow, purple, orange and red. This week we'll add another serving of fruits and/or vegetables to your daily diet to move closer to the Food Guide Pyramid. By now you should be changing your focus from meats, fats and refined sugar to starches, vegetables and fruits.

One of my favorite ways to get an extra portion of vegetables is to have a plate of vegetable munchies before dinner. Prior to starting dinner, put out a tray of peeled carrots, celery, peppers, cucumbers, pickles, cherry tomatoes, orange sections, grapes, berries or whatever you like. Often, this is the main source of vegetables for my children. If I put it before them when they are hungry, they will eat it. If I wait until dinner is served, they go for the meat and starch first and then it is a chore to get them to eat the vegetables. Avoid dips, just go for the plain vegetables. This will also give you something to munch on while fixing dinner, rather than sampling the more fattening items.

Of course, a great salad is the perfect way to add vegetables to your diet. Experiment with a variety of red and green lettuces. Romaine, Boston, bibb, spinach and leaf lettuce are more nutrient-rich than the classic iceberg head-lettuce.

Fruit salad makes a great first course. Avoid canned fruit which is usually packed in syrup. Choose ripe fruits in great colors, such as an orange melon, red strawberry, blueberry and green kiwi fruit. With their gorgeous colors a fruit salad is hard to resist.

A piece of fruit can also put a nice finishing touch on a meal. A fruit salad can be a substitute for a high-calorie dessert. When you have finished your meal, top it off with an orange. An orange not only cleanses your palate, but also cleans the air with that wonderful scent. Ambrosia makes a great dessert—orange or tangerine sections and grapes sprinkled with shredded coconut.

Try adding a fruit to your breakfast, either alone or on cereal or yogurt.

Another way to add a fruit or vegetable serving per day is with a glass of juice. An added benefit to this is that many orange juices are now fortified with calcium. When purchasing fruit juices, insist on 100% fruit juice. The best way to control the content of juices is to make your own.

# WEEK 29: THE HEALTHY KITCHEN

No doubt your kitchen could use an overhaul. You may have acquired years of poor cooking habits and endless array of appliances that scream out "use me!" Your kitchen and cooking methods should reflect your new healthy lifestyle. For starters, no one who is serious about their health and weight should keep a deep fryer in their home. Breaded and fried items are especially high in fat because the breading soaks up the fat. If you have a fryer, give it away. If it remains in the kitchen, it will be too much of a temptation to resist. If you must have deep fried items, you can have them once a month at a restaurant (choose one that uses vegetable oils to fry, not lard.) By now, however, your taste for high-fat foods should have diminished.

Here are some appliances for a well-equipped healthy kitchen:

- An outdoor grill is a must. You can grill almost any meat and/or vegetable. Grilled shishkabobs are a great meal. Skewer bite size pieces of chicken or shellfish, with lots of vegetables such as peppers, onions, mushrooms, yellow squash, zucchini, etc. Serve over rice or pasta. Almost any grilled fish makes a good low-fat meal also. You don't need an elaborate grill. A simple charcoal grill will produce a taste every bit as good as the huge, multi-gadget, multi-burner grill. The medium that you use to keep heat will make a difference in flavor, and experimentation is worth the effort. Mesquite chips, hickory chips, lava rocks, and charcoals will impart different flavors and aromas to the food.

- A kitchen scale. You should weigh your portions often until you are very good at estimation. Then, weigh periodically to keep yourself in check.

- A steamer for vegetables. This does not have to be a separate appliance. A simple metal basket that fits inside a pot with a lid is ideal. The basket keeps the vegetables out of the water and they are cooked by the rising steam. Steaming, rather than boiling, retains more vitamins in the vegetables. They should be cooked until just tender, not overcooked. If you don't have a steamer, you can use a pan with a tightly fitting lid and just cover the bottom of the pan with about and inch of water. No oil, butter or margarine is needed.

- A gravy separator. This is a cup with a spout that comes out from the bottom. Liquids will separate with the fat on the top, allowing you to pour off the low-fat liquid at the bottom for gravies and sauces. You can then discard the fat. If you parboil chicken, you can pour the stock into a gravy separator. Let cool. You can then pour the flavorful stock into another container, leaving the fat at the top. You can use this same method for separating the fat from pan drippings prior to making gravy.

- Non-stick pans. The new non-stick pans are much improved and used by some of the greatest chefs in the world. Utensils will not scratch them, and browning is improved.

Get a good quality pan, and you can eliminate your need for cooking oil.

- A bread machine. Low-fat bread fresh from a bread maker is wonderful, without butter or spreads.

- A salad spinner. This inexpensive, ingenious plastic invention will insure that your salad greens are clean and dry. It is a plastic colander which fits inside another plastic bowl. The top contains a gear driven handle which spins the inside colander so fast that water is thrown off the greens by centrifugal force. Works like a charm. It is also a good way to store greens.

- Good containers for dispensing: a spray bottle for vinegars and salad dressings with no solids; a pump bottle such as a hand soap bottle for thicker dressings; and a shaker for powdered sugar and granulated sugar. These will give you much better coverage while using less.

- An air–popper for popcorn. Popcorn is a great low–fat snack when popped without oil. You can get either a countertop unit, or a microwave popper.

- A pressure cooker. Dried beans are nutritious, filling and the perfect staple for the low–fat pantry. However, they can take hours to cook on the stove. A pressure cooker can cut this time to minutes.

Take a serious look through your kitchen. It should help and not hinder your new lifestyle. If you are an avid baker, you may have to make some difficult choices. But these choices made now will be easier than resisting the temptation time and time again in the future.

# Week 30: Unfinished Business

**M**uch like making a list of fun things last quarter, this week make a list of things to do instead of eating. Undoubtedly there are dozens of things that could be done around your home, with your career, your family and your education—chores, obligations, repairs and unfinished business. List them all, and when boredom strikes, grab your list and check one off. Not only will you resist the urge to overeat, you will also improve your environment and relationships. For example:

- Paint a room
- Change the oil in the car
- Clean out a closet
- Organize your receipts to make tax time easier
- Give the dog a bath
- Reline the kitchen cabinets
- Clean out the refrigerator
- Write a letter to an old friend
- Review your child's homework

- Visit an elderly relative
- Do some household repairs for an elderly or disabled relative or neighbor
- Learn how to use a computer program
- Research your family genealogy
- Take a CPR or first aid class
- Repot or propagate your indoor plants
- Change the furnace filter
- Make a will
- Balance your checkbook
- Clean the windows
- Get out those "thin" clothes and iron them, or alter some of your "fat" clothes.
- Shampoo the carpet
- Wash and wax your car
- If it's winter, dig up your flower bulbs and split them. Give away half to neighbors and friends.
- Clean your gutters
- Get a haircut

Using the following To-Do List, make your own list. As you move through this week, look at your environment with a critical eye and list anything that you can to improve it. Next time you are hungry and in danger of overeating, grab your To-Do List and get started.

# To-Do List

# WEEK 31: GROWING GROCERIES

P lease give this serious consideration before deciding that gardening is not for you. I put "gardening" in several places in the *Live It!* Plan book before realizing that it deserves an entire chapter and week of consideration. It could easily be just another activity or exercise, or tip to increase the amount of produce in your diet. I realized it is far too important to tuck away and should be considered by everyone who is serious about weight loss and eating healthy. Here's why:

- You get the best tasting and freshest produce from a garden. Produce from the market is at best two days old and usually far older. It has suffered through transportation and unknown climate fluctuations while in transit. In fact, most of the produce in markets is from other countries or states and often has been sprayed with chemicals to stave off ripening during shipment and then to induce ripening once it hits the store shelves. Many varieties of supermarket produce are selected for their endurance during transportation, shelf life and looks, NOT taste. If you have never had produce directly from a garden, you will be amazed at the difference in taste. Improve your odds of liking fruits and vegetables by eating the best.

- Gardening puts you in complete control of the herbicides and pesticides that you ingest. How do you know what chemicals are used in the fruit you eat? With fruit coming from all over the world, how can you be sure that they use safe levels of chemicals? More and more research shows that chemicals are not needed to provide an ample harvest. Crop rotation, natural insect predators (fire ants are my favorite), companion planting, hand weeding and many more efforts can easily produce great harvests without the use of pesticides and herbicides.

- Tending to a garden and spending a good deal of time with it will increase your odds of making fruits and vegetables a central focus of your diet. Vegetables will be more in your thoughts. Rather than reading dessert cookbooks, you will be reading seed catalogs and vegetable cookbooks.

- Gardening is a wonderful means of exercise. It can be light, such as simple weeding or planting seeds, or it can be quite vigorous, such as plowing and turning the soil. Gardening is a great activity for all ages. Children love a garden. Even the very elderly can tend to a modest garden.

- Gardening is stress reducing.

"I see the benefits, but", you say...


**I don't have a piece of property.** Even if you live in an apartment, you can garden. Herb gardens can be grown indoors almost anywhere. If you don't even have a window with good light you can get a grow light. There are mail-order catalogs devoted to hydroponic gardening.

You can barter with someone who does have a piece of property. Offer them a portion of your produce, or offer to clear a portion of their land in exchange for a year or two of leasing. They'll probably be delighted that their land will be cultivated.

Approach a city or county government and offer to cultivate a vacant piece of property. Start with your local county extension agent. Not only can they help you find a place to garden, they will also have valuable advice on growing tips for your climate. Many state agricultural departments have a free publication. In Georgia, it is called the Market Bulletin. A subscription is free, and you can place a free ad inquiring about garden space. If you find a big enough piece of property, find a few others and start a coop. Many land owners would be more than happy to have someone care for their property and keep it cultivated.

Approach a local retirement home, private school, or day care center. Offer to start a garden club for the elderly or the children.

You really don't have to own a huge piece of property to garden. You can have a very prolific garden in a 12 foot by 12 foot plot. Read *Square Foot Gardening* by Mel Barthalomew.

**It's winter. Nothing will grow in the winter. It's the dead of summer. Nothing can be started now.** Gardening is a year round activity. If it's February and you have two more months of frost, it's time to consult your gardening catalogs and start your seeds indoors. This will give you a jump on the season. If it's the dead of summer, just pay more attention to watering and weeding. No matter what time of year it is, you can be researching, planning the garden or shopping for supplies.

**I live in the North and there's just a tiny growing season.** There are hotbeds and green houses to extend the growing seasons in colder climates. Just watch the "Victory Garden" on a Public Broadcasting station and see how productive a New England garden can be.

**I'm too old.** No one is too old or too young to garden. You may need raised beds that you can work at while sitting, or you can work in a greenhouse. You can ask your support partner, a child or teenager in your area to help with the heavier work.

**I have a bad back.** If you have a bad back, your overweight condition is most certainly an aggravating factor. There are excellent references that teach back strengthening exercises and prevention methods. There are wonderful back braces now on the market. See your medical doctor or chiropractor for more information.

**I just don't like gardening.** If you've put the right amount of effort into gardening, it's hard not to love it. If you have had a complete season and properly tended to your plants, the outcome will be wonderful food, and a great sense of accomplishment. It is only natural for humans to love cultivating plants.

**It's too expensive.** It doesn't have to be expensive. Plant twice as much as you will eat and sell the remainder. A local gardening club or your County Extension Agent can help you maintain a very cost effective garden. Many counties also maintain canning facilities that you can use to preserve your surplus for the off season months. You can share equipment and buy supplies and seeds in bulk with another gardener. It doesn't have to be expensive and if done efficiently, can reduce your food bill.

**I don't have the time.** With so many things tugging at our attention throughout the day, this can be understandable. However, how many hours per day do you watch TV? You say you need that to unwind? Try gardening. It can be the most relaxing and refreshing activity of all. Spend an hour of "quality time" with your kids in the garden. They will love to be involved. Use your lunch hour, twice a week. Be creative and make gardening one of your priorities.

**I just don't think it will be successful.** Your garden will produce if you tend to it consistently. Start small, with one or two varieties and learn everything you can about those. Visit your garden regularly, at least once a week. Examine your plants and remedy what ails them before it gets out of control. Pull the weeds before they take over. Spray the aphids with dilute soapy water before they eat up half of your harvest. If you see something you can't identify, call your County Extension Agent or consult the library or local nursery. Be observant and *tend* your garden. Your success will be directly and clearly related to the time and attention you devote.

A great way to get started gardening is to offer to help a neighbor who already keeps a successful garden. While you provide some of the work, they can provide valuable experience that is specifically for your climate, soil and pests. Ask for a share of the harvest in return for your work.

I hope I've convinced you to start a garden. Whether it's for herbs, mushrooms, annual vegetables, grape vines, a fruit or nut orchard, or berry bushes, I truly think you will enjoy it. This year, you are refocusing your life. Gardening can help you do this.

# WEEK 32: TAME YOUR SWEET TOOTH

**M**ost American diets include too much refined sugar. The problem with refined sugar is that it is too highly concentrated in calories, and contains practically no nutrients. All this does is add excess calories to your diet, and make you more prone to obesity and diabetes.

Americans eat an average of 70 pounds per year of sugar. Sugar is not only found in an abundance of sweet treats, but also in many processed foods as preservatives, thickeners or baking aids.

*How easy it is for those*
*Who do not bulge*
*To not overindulge!*
*- Ogden Nash*

Foods that contain one of the following as the first or second ingredient are likely to be high in sugar: brown sugar, corn sweetener, corn syrup, fructose, fruit juice concentrate, glucose (dextrose), high-fructose corn syrup, honey, invert sugar, lactose, maltose, molasses, raw sugar, table sugar (sucrose) or syrup.

Reducing sugar in your diet is logical for health and weight loss, but to those with a sweet tooth, it's a tough pill to swallow. As we have said in past weeks, you should not be denied all the foods you love. But you must be realistic and keep moderation in mind. In the last several months you have learned many tricks for dealing with other problem foods. More importantly, you have gained control and the self confidence that you can do this. The choice is yours. Consider the following to reduce your intake of refined sugar:

1.  Reduce the number of times that you indulge. Do you eat candy bars every day? Twice a day? Limit yourself to one every other day, and then, in three months, drop that to two per week. If that sweet tooth really nags, chew a piece of gum or slowly dissolve a piece of hard candy. This might be all you need.

2.  Make a better choice. Try fruit dipped in powdered or brown sugar, frozen fruit sticks or just orange juice frozen in popsicle trays. Try a low-fat pudding or custard with berries. Jell–O, vanilla wafers, a lollipop or butterscotch are also good choices. Many sweets are not only heavy with sugar, but also fat, such as cheesecake, ice cream, chocolate candy bars and donuts. These are the ones to avoid.

3.  Eat a reduced calorie version. Reduced calorie brands are not always palatable, and some are much better than others. Try a couple different brands and varieties and find one that suits your particular taste. I tend to avoid excess artificial sweeteners and artificial fat because they can produce side effects. Many people tend to overeat reduced calorie items, and end up eating more calories than are in a reasonable portion of the real thing. Also, note that many items that are reduced fat have added sugar. When baking, try to reduce the amount of sugar, chocolate, oil and nuts. Applesauce can replace most or all of the oil required in a recipe.

4. Eat smaller portions. Measure your serving. What you think is one half cup might turn out to be a cup and a half. Share a restaurant dessert with someone at the table. Cut your candy bar in half and save half for later. Get a single scoop of ice cream. Avoid purchasing a large bag of candy, or an entire cake or pie. If you bake, bake cupcakes rather than a large cake.

Decide which way is the best and easiest way for you to reduce the number of calories you consume from refined sugars. Experiment until you have control. Perhaps a combination of two of the above methods works best for you. This week, work on one particular item, such as that mid-morning candy bar, and then in three months, tackle another.

# WEEK 33: MOVE IT AND LOSE IT

L ast quarter you chose an activity and by now you should be devoting at least 60 minutes per week at that activity. This week, double this to a total of 120 minutes each week. That can be 30 minutes on 4 days, or 20 minutes on 6 days. Check with your healthcare professional to insure that this level of activity is safe for you.

It is particularly important to become involved in a *regularly occurring* activity. You want to form a habit, and develop a mindset and metabolism that expects regular exercise. You may want to choose two or three different activities. For instance, coach a soccer team on Tuesday and Thursday evenings, walk with your child or a friend on Thursday and volunteer to help build a Habit for Humanity house on the weekend. This will tone different sets of muscles and give your body a well rounded workout, without the boredom of a regimented exercise routine.

You may not think of yourself as an active or athletic person, but this is a mindset that is important to develop. Your exercise and activity should never be considered a "chore" or "obligation". If it is, something needs to change. Concentrate on changing your attitude towards activity. Enjoy the fresh air and sunshine. Anticipate how great you'll feel for accomplishing something that will bring you closer to your goal.

For an otherwise healthy individual, experts recommend one half to one hour of exercise at least three times per week, preferably on all days of the week. We'll work up to that goal by the end of the year.

# WEEK 34: CELEBRATE!

P arties and holidays are time for celebration and joy, but all too often add to our temptations. Since you may have started the Live It! Plan at any time during the year, this week many not coincide with a holiday. You may want to swap this week for a holiday week in the future.

The average American gains four to six pounds during the year end holidays. Entire industries revolve around this fact; food merchants such as caterers and grocery stores boom during this time. It always amazes me how crowded the market is just before a holiday. On the other hand, weight management programs, athletic clubs and exercise equipment boom in January. Just watch the advertisements. Don't get caught in that trap. Here are some ways to avoid overindulgence during holidays:

> *Concentrate on the event at hand rather than the food. Thanksgiving is as much about friendship, sharing, life and health, as it is about an abundance of food.*

- If you are hosting an event and guests ask what they can bring, request flowers, a candle or an ornament rather than another dessert.

- If you have more than one home to visit on a holiday, start alternating one this year and one the next year. Never try to attend two holiday meals in one day. You will feel obligated to eat both meals.

- After dinner, rather than falling asleep in front of the TV, take a walk with several guests.

- Don't ever hesitate to decline the offer for an extra helping, dessert or appetizer. This is not an insult and should not be received as one. Compliment the cook and say that dinner was excellent and more than enough.

- Send the leftovers home with the guests. I tend to cook entirely too much, especially for large family meals. However, many guests love to take sliced turkey or lasagna home for a meal the next day. Throughout the year, I save plastic containers or jars, such as those from yogurt and cottage cheese. These come in handy to fill with leftovers, and the guests do not have to worry about returning the containers.

- Plan in your food journal, and stick to it. If you don't know what will be served, generalize. Promise to avoid the appetizers, refuse second helpings, or control your dessert portion. Being mentally prepared is a powerful tool in controlling your diet. Believe it and use it.

- Eat healthy and light the week before and the week after.

- Wear slightly snug pants so you can feel tightness before overeating.

- Do you love to bake for a holiday? Bake dough ornaments or an herb bread wreath instead of cookies and pies.

- Rather than a pie, bake a fruit crisp. Very often most of the fat grams in a pie are in the crust. Avoid pecan pie, chocolate pie and cheesecake. Better yet, serve fresh berries dipped in brown sugar or powdered sugar.

- Cook a turkey breast rather than a whole turkey. Not only will you have only lean white meat, but also the gravy that you make from baking a breast will be much leaner. You can buy a whole turkey breast, on the bone either frozen or fresh. I find that the boneless turkey breasts do not taste nearly as good as those with the bone. I cannot taste a difference between the fresh and frozen, so I often keep a frozen turkey breast on hand.

- Have appetizers of vegetables and fruit. Try a dip with a yogurt or salsa base.

- Concentrate on the event at hand rather than the food. Thanksgiving is as much about friendship, sharing, life and health, as it is about an abundance of food. And of course, the spiritual intent of many holidays is often lost in the exchange of gifts and elaborate display of food. Enjoy your holiday and party. Enjoy great conversations and concentrate on the celebration.

# WEEK 35: AFTERNOON SNACKING

We've worked on breakfast, mid-morning and lunch. By now you should be starting your day off right. Why ruin a good start to the day? That mid-afternoon hour is the next to tackle. If you have no problems with overeating during this time of the day, use this week to sharpen your skills that were learned in previous weeks.

The afternoon is the perfect time for diversions and errands. Stores and businesses are open, the sun is high in the sky for outdoor activities, and most people are out and about. What is your afternoon snacking pattern? Does it hit at about two o'clock and not stop until dinner? Looks like two o'clock would be a good time to schedule an activity—call on a customer or neighbor, take care of your garden or play a game with the kids. If this is the time of the day when you overeat the most, schedule your regular activity during this time.

> *By, God, Mr. Chairman, at this moment I stand astonished at my own moderation!*
> *– Robert, Lord Clive*

Try a diversion. Consult your List of Fun Things, your To-Do List, or try one of these:

- Make a phone call to a chatty friend.

- Recite your goal.

- Ask yourself, "if I eat this, how long will it taste good, and then how long will I feel bad for eating it? Is it worth the consequences?"

- Call your support partner.

- Write it down. Describe why you want to eat, and how you will feel if you eat, and how you will feel if you don't.

- Chew a piece of gum.

- Brush your teeth.

Look back into your food journal and see on average how many calories you are consuming between lunch and dinner. Starting today, cut that back by one half. If you have been eating 500 calories, cut it back to 250. Then, move ahead a few months and make a note to cut back to 150 calories. Try to put off the snack as long as you can. If you can wait until 30 to 45 minutes before dinner, it will decrease your appetite for dinner. Review the snack list in Week 5: The Mid-Morning Hours.

You may want to resolve never to buy from a snack machine again. They are too expensive, and almost always a smorgasbord of poor choices. Don't even look at them. Don't keep change in your wallet or drawer. If you've done your planning, there is no reason to buy anything from a snack machine.

# WEEK 36: LOOSEN UP AND CHILL OUT

S tress can be a major factor contributing to overeating but it can be controlled. When things get absolutely crazy, don't compound your stress by overeating or by taking it out on those around you. In addition to overeating, stress can cause stomach cramps, loose bowels, insomnia, increased blood pressure, poor judgement and rash reactions, inability to concentrate, backaches, irritability, increased smoking and alcohol abuse. Recognize the stress for what it is and try one of these:

- Identify the source of your stress and make a change where possible.

- Leave enough time for yourself to get ready and meet appointments. Allow time for traffic. If you are one of those incurable late arrivers, set your clocks ahead. This wouldn't fool me, but it does seem to help some folks. If it's your spouse or child that is always late, tell them that the appointment is 15 or 30 minutes earlier than it really is.

- Spend 15 minutes every day to schedule your time. You can do this at the same time you fill out your food journal plan. If you are a very busy person, get a time organizer and learn how to use it. Having a small notebook (you can also adapt your food journal for this use) closeby to jot down important numbers, dates, ideas or to-dos is a great stress reliever. Use it to jot down things you need from the store when it comes to mind. Get those important and nagging details down on paper. You can then free your mind knowing that those important facts can be retrieved

> *When angry, count to four; when very angry, swear.*
> *- Mark Twain*

reliably at any time, by just referring to your notebook. The key to making a time organizer work is to keep it with you at all times.

- Count to ten or take a short walk before acting in a stressful situation. Delay your reaction until you can process all the facts, and calmly respond. A poorly contrived, impulsive response to a stressful situation can often compound the problem.

- Compromise. Give in occasionally. Let someone in front of you in a traffic jam. Let your spouse have the last word.

- Laugh. Find a book of jokes and keep it handy. Opt for a comedy movie. Listen to comedy tapes

> *For fast acting relief, try slowing down. -Lily Tomlin*

in the car. Laugh out loud, and laugh at yourself. Be quick to smile and find humor in any situation.

- Put your keys, purse and wallet in the same location every day.

- Make sure you have duplicates of any item that would be painful to lose, such as car keys, house keys, computer files, etc. Keep the duplicates in a safe, accessible place. Photocopies of certain documents and credit card numbers can make replacement easier.

- Pay attention to nutrition. A proper diet, as you are achieving, will help you lose weight and reduce stress.

- Walk or exercise. This is a proven stress reliever and cannot be over emphasized as a key element of a healthy lifestyle. You can also use your time during walking to plan or reinforce your short term and long term goals.

- Reduce or eliminate caffeine. Caffeine can contribute to mood swings, irritability and insomnia.

- Realize that some things are not under your control. Tackle those that you can change, but let go of the ones that you cannot influence.

- Worrying can be obsessive and consuming. It is not only ineffective, but damaging to your psyche and your relationships. Many people bring stress upon themselves while worrying about things that will never happen, or things that are beyond their control. Worrying is an assumption that an outcome will be negative. Why not assume that the outcome will be bright and positive? Your attitude may, in fact, influence the outcome.

- Lay out clothes for yourself and the kids each night for the next day. If you can, prepare several days clothes in advance.

- For those items that you can't do without and which are not perishable, keep an ample supply. There's no reason why you shouldn't have an extra anti-perspirant, plenty of underwear or an extra box of laundry detergent on hand.

- Avoid traffic. Change your hours at work or your route to work. Avoid making appointments which will take you into heavy traffic.

- Never let your gas tank get below a quarter of a tank. You do not want to be running out of gas *and* be late for an appointment.

- Learn to say "No" to excessive commitments. Care for yourself and your family first. Take on only those things that you can accomplish well, without sacrificing your sanity.

- Don't even look at your junk mail or catalogs. Stand over the trashcan and deal your mail like a deck of cards. Better yet, take the time to send a note to catalog companies that you do not use. They don't want to waste mailings to people who are not interested.

- Get a stress management tape or book. Learn relaxation techniques.

- Missing a birthday or having to buy a card or gift at the last minute can be stressing. Next time you are in the card section of the store, browse for several minutes and pick up several cards for birthdays in the coming months. If you have small children, keep a wrapped toy on hand to send to a birthday party.

- Take a class on Yoga or meditation.

- Don't procrastinate. If there is something you need to do, just do it. You will feel relief that it is done, rather than the anxiety of a deadline. There are many excellent audio tapes and books available to help the procrastinator.

- Build a fire in the fireplace.

- Listen to some great music.

- Don't buy uncomfortable shoes. The last thing you need nagging at you is your feet.

- Play with your pet. Get an aquarium.

- Make your lunches or kids lunches as far in advance as you can. Pack up five lunches with the non-perishables and just add the perishables each morning.

- Unplug your telephone and read for a couple hours.

- Give your kids a hug and kiss.

- Pay for some household help once a week or month.

- Lay down in a quiet spot for five minutes.

- Get a massage or a facial.

There are many things you can do to control stress. Anticipate stressful situations and plan to avoid them. It's all a matter of control. You should be well on your way to controlling your diet, and stress is just one more aspect of life in which planning and control can play a major role.

# WEEK 37: SHAVE THE CRAVE

V ery often, an overeater has one or two really challenging problem foods or categories of foods. These not only add most of the extra unneeded calories to your daily diet, but they also haunt you and tempt you and chip away at your resolve to eat better. One binge with a potato chip bag can put a damper on the best laid eating plans. Guilt takes over, and your attitude changes to "Well, to-day's wasted." Taking control of these problem areas will give you great satisfaction.

*No problem is so big and complicated that it can't be run away from.*
*-Linus, Charles Schultz*

Now is when you might think "This is where I fail. I can't live without chocolate." Slow down. Take a deep breath. You don't have to live without your favorite food. In fact, depriving yourself of your favorite foods can lead to cravings and binge eating. The key is control and moderation. We are going to tackle this slowly and methodically, just as we have been all along. Our goal is to change the *cravings* that drive you into overeating, and gradually change a problem food into an occasional treat without the guilt.

Let's examine an effective plan to do this:

1. Identify the problem area. Is it a particular food such as chocolate, or is it a whole class of foods such as fried salty snacks? Is it one particular restaurant? You probably know immediately what it is. If not, look back into your food journal.

2. Dissect the circumstances that bring on the cravings. You have been building valuable research data every day as you record what you eat. Since you have been recording what you eat, see at what time you eat this particular item. Is it always between nine and ten o'clock in the evening? Is it only after you've skipped a meal? Is it Friday evenings? During your favorite TV show? After a fight with your spouse? After a bad day at work? Think back and try to spot a pattern that leads to triggering the craving for this food. Use this ammunition to build a plan to avoid those circumstances, or deal with them in another way.

3. Build your plan to take control of this problem food. You have developed tools and skills to make this work. Use your food journal to record reminders. Here is how to start: avoid the onset of the craving. Don't put yourself in the same circumstances that lead to the craving. If your problem is from nine to ten while watching TV, plan to read in another room during that time. Take yourself out of the scene that triggers the overeating. Avoid the restaurant. Don't skip a meal. Be proactive in avoiding stress. Stay active.

Grab your "List of Fun Things To Do" or your "To-Do List." If you can put off the craving for even one half an hour, you may very well be able to put it out of your mind completely.

You don't have to eliminate your favorite food forever. But if you don't get it under control, you will never be able to truly enjoy it. Have a smaller portion, have it less often, and/or reduce the caloric content.

Try not to reach for a high-calorie treat on an empty stomach. Save that chocolate for after a meal. You will be much more likely to eat moderately if your appetite has been satisfied by a good, healthy meal.

Make the process of eating the problem food difficult. Don't keep the food in the house. Lose the phone number to the pizza delivery place. Review the chapter "Set the Stage for Success." Spend this week pinpointing your most difficult challenge and the circumstances that set you up for overeating. Chip away at it day by day, incident by incident.

If you do occasionally break down and overindulge, promise to do better the next time. Get right back on track, that very day. There is no benefit in being excessively hard on yourself for a lack of control. Don't beat yourself up. Simply recognize that this act is keeping you from your goal. Learn from the incident. Learn more about why it happens and what you might do in the future to avoid it or lessen the severity.

Next quarter we will take another approach to increase your control over these problem areas.

# WEEK 38: GO FISH

F ish and seafood are an excellent source of low-fat protein. Many American diets do not include fish. One of the seven dietary guidelines is to eat a variety of foods, and you can do this easily with fish. Even land-locked states now have fresh fish readily available, and many vacuum sealed frozen filets are excellent. Fresh, filleted (boneless) fish is best, and don't be afraid to spend a bit per pound more than you would on meat. Most fish and seafood have very little waste. You won't be paying for bones and fat that you will discard, so often the price per pound ends up no higher than a good cut of meat after cooking. Give yourself the best possible chance to love fish and seafood by buying the best cuts.

Visit a large seafood market and try some of the variety that is available. Try different shellfish such as scallops, lobster, langostinos, prawns, crab, oysters and shrimp. The variety of fresh water and saltwater filleted fish is astounding. Choose one. If you find you don't care for the taste, be sure to try another. Fish can be flaky or dense, bland or strong, white or dark, and tough or tender. One variety might be best for soups, while another best for grilling. So be sure to try several varieties, cooked in several ways. The people at the market should be able to provide cooking instructions and may even have sample recipe handouts. Use these guidelines when selecting and preparing fish and seafood:

- Avoid fried fish, especially breaded and fried. Opt for stewed, baked, grilled, blackened, poached or steamed.

- Always opt for albacore tuna packed in water rather than oil. To remove all the water after opening the can, I squeeze the lid onto the tuna, then place the tuna on two folded sheets of paper towels in a covered plastic container. Refrigerate for an hour or so, and most of the water will be absorbed by the paper towels. Albacore costs a little more, but the difference in taste and smell is well worth it. Tuna sprinkled on a pasta or green salad makes a wonderful meal. A can of tuna in the pantry makes a great last minute meal. If you like tuna salad, try a sandwich with a spread of mayonnaise, a bed of lettuce or sprouts and the flaked tuna. You will use much less mayonnaise if you spread a bit on the bread rather than mixing it in with the tuna.

- Avoid the most expensive salmon which is high in fat. Lower priced salmon will be more lean. Sea bass also has a high-fat content relative to many other cuts.

- Fresh fish and seafood should be either frozen or cooked the day of purchase.

- Avoid smoked whole fish which is high in oils.

- Try fish chowders, gumbos and stews, with a vegetable base rather than a cream base.

- Avoid fried fish sandwiches which can have just as much fat (or more) as a cheeseburger.

- Avoid fish sticks and frozen prepared fish entrees. Most are ground fish and are high in fats and salt. Frozen popcorn shrimp are usually nothing more that tiny bits of shrimp with a heavy coating of breading soaked in oil.

- Serve a tomato based cocktail sauce rather than tartar sauce with fish.

- If bones in a filet turn you off, choose a filet from a large salt water fish such as Mahi Mahi or marlin. Smaller fish will have tiny bones down the spine which are nearly impossible to remove completely.

- Invest in a seafood and fish cookbook and guide.

Phase fish into your diet so that by the end of the year you have two meals based on fish or seafood per week. If fish has never been a part of your diet, it may take you a while to acquire a taste. But once you have, you will find it a welcome addition.

# WEEK 39: THIRD QUARTER REVIEW

Y ou are three quarters of the way to lifelong weight control. If you have used your food journal, adopted each weekly change, and are using most of the tips, you are most definitely on the way. You have established a strong foundation of habits and eating patterns that will help you continue to lose weight. You should have a solid knowledge of nutrition, how to calculate portions, and the calorie and fat content of most of the foods you eat. This is the week to review your progress and goals and adjust as necessary.

At times, you may have felt deprived or unsatisfied. You may find it hard to push yourself to increase your physical activity. Regard these as *temporary indications that you are moving towards your goal.* They will subside and go away. These feelings are as temporary as the feeling of satisfaction that you get from overeating. If you are feeling overly deprived, perhaps you are trying to lose too much weight and adjust to new healthy habits too quickly.

Review your original weight loss goals. If you feel obsessed with certain problem foods, or food in general, you may be pushing your body and metabolism to change too rapidly. Your chances of keeping weight off are much greater when you lose it slowly, while building solid nutritional habits. Settle in, and acknowledge that your life is changing, slowly and surely. As long as you see a downward trend, even if it is very gradual, you are on the right track.

Review your food journal to see where you can improve. Zero in on one problem spot and analyze it. Is it the time between breakfast and lunch? Is it the morning donuts? Fear of vegetables? After dinner runs to the ice cream shop? Your route past the tempting fast food window? Stress? What tiny steps can you take, week by week to gradually correct this, to chip away at the problem, to gain control?

> *Slight not what's near, when aiming at what's far. -Euripides*

Review each of the weeks in this quarter and list one more thing you can do to reinforce the task of the week. Here are some suggestions:

**Let's Do Lunch:** Once a week, have a carton of yogurt and read a classic novel for lunch.

**Good Things Are Green:** Try a spaghetti squash with to-mato sauce for dinner tonight.

**The Healthy Kitchen:** Get smaller serving dishes and serv-ing spoons.

**Unfinished Business:** Make a separate To-Do list for the of-fice.

*Growing Groceries:* Look up a gardening show on TV and plan to watch it this week, or get a gardening video at the library.

*Tame Your Sweet Tooth:* Put some table sugar in a salt shaker and shake it on berries and cereal rather than spooning on.

*Move It and Lose It:* If you break up your exercise into small time slots, get a stop watch and keep a running total of your minutes.

*Celebrate!:* Write a reminder in your food journal just before each holiday to review this chapter.

*Afternoon Snacking:* Replace the afternoon snacking habit with another habit such as reading the newspaper or searching the Internet.

*Loosen Up and Chill Out:* Go to bed one half hour earlier and get up one half hour earlier. Give yourself more time in the morning to arrange the day.

*Shave The Crave:* Use a highlighter to mark the occurrences of a problem food in your food journal. This will make it easier for you to spot a pattern.

*Go Fish:* Try a clam bake for an outdoor party rather than meat on the grill.

You are building resolve, confidence, self control, self esteem and a solid foundation for years of healthy living. There are still three more months packed with great methods and tips to help drop your weight even further.

# FOURTH

# QUARTER:

# FINISHING

# TOUCHES

# WEEK 40: DINNER

For most Americans, dinner is the largest meal of the day. It is also more than just a meal—it is a social event, and a time for the family to touch base and gather together. This can also be the one meal of the day that is not rushed and that can be well planned and nutritionally sound. You have come a long way, and learned many skills to manage your diet. It's time to apply these skills to the dinner hour.

As mentioned in week 27, "Let's Do Lunch", if this meal is your primary meal, you may find it very difficult to reduce severely. Everyone has unique tastes, appetites and challenges. Structure your plan for moderating your diet with success in mind. Reduce more gradually if dinner is especially satisfying for you. Reduce quicker if you are normally not very hungry at that hour.

Try one or more of these ideas:

- Have your afternoon snack as late in the day as possible to cut your hunger before dinner.

- Take a brisk walk before dinner.

- Get into the habit of serving a "de-appetizer" 15 minutes before the meal, such as broth based soup, salad, raw vegetables, or fruit. This way you will be more apt to eat the nutritional foods first while you are hungry, and it will cut your appetite for the more fattening entree.

- Beware of the effects of alcohol. It not only adds non-nutritional calories to your diet, but also lessens your resolve and self discipline.

- Your dinner hour can be difficult if you have family members who are not interested in eating healthy. Usually, if the cook is eating healthy, so is the rest of the household. If you're the cook, you're in control. If not, your offer to cook may be enthusiastically welcomed. However, this is just like a smoker trying to quit when their spouse does not. It can create stress for all family members. Promise to keep your commitment to yourself, and set an example for others at the table. It may be tough at first, but your success and attitude can be contagious.

  *Never eat anything at one sitting that you can't lift.*
  *-Miss Piggy*
  *(Jim Henson/Frank Oz)*

- Distract yourself so you don't over-sample while cooking. Turn on the radio while making dinner, or have a "How was your day?" conversation with a family member.

- Chew gum while making dinner. This will help you avoid picking and taste testing. Ten taste tests before dinner can easily add up to an entire serving. And, this type of grazing is extremely difficult to quantify in your food journal.

- Rather than ending dinner with a sugary dessert, try fruit dipped in brown sugar or powdered sugar, cup of hot spiced tea, sugar-free gelatin, or frozen orange juice popsicle.

- Make family conversation a major focus of the dinner hour. Use this time to reconnect with your children, and/or mate. Talk about the day and plans for tomorrow.

- Take a brisk walk after dinner.

- After a good day and a satisfying dinner, plan for tomorrow's meals. Get your food journal out and make some commitments.

*If you wish to grow thinner, diminish your dinner.*
*- H. S. Leigh*

As always, just because you are cutting down your consumption during the dinner hour, be careful that you are not compensating for this by adding calories at other times of the day. Monitor this in your food journal.

# WEEK 41: BRING ON THE BREAD

I t's time once again to focus on starches as the basis of your diet. If you are not already eating six to eleven servings per day (depending on your body frame size), then this week add another one or two servings per day. If you already have enough starches, try making some more nutritious choices. Here are some more ways to get the most out of starches in your diet:

*Breads*. Consider a bread machine. These wonderful appliances really do work. You simply put the ingredients in, one on top of the other, shut the top and turn it on. In three to four hours you have a great tasting homemade loaf of bread with no preservatives. Bread just out of the oven is fabulous without added toppings such as butter. Even though it is relatively fat-free, you may have to restrain yourself from eating half the loaf. You also get the benefit of the wonderful aroma of baking bread. The popularity of these machines has spawned hundreds of great recipe books. You can also buy bread mixes that only require liquid ingredients and the yeast. Experiment with less refined flours such as whole wheat, rye, and oat, both when you are baking bread and buying bread.

**Rices.** Try the less refined rices such as brown and wild, or another variety of rice such as basmati, jasmine or nikishi. Try rice cakes for one of your daily snacks. Cooked, cooled white rice, pressed into a pie pan, makes a great base for a quiche, and replaces a high-fat pie crust.

**Pastas.** Try fresh pastas rather than dried. Either make your own or buy in the deli section of your grocery store. Try wheat pastas. Spinach and tomato varieties make a beautiful cold pasta salad. Look for couscous which is a tasty, tiny pasta common in Middle Eastern countries that cooks in five minutes. You can find it usually near the rice section. Many mixes are available that include spices.

**Whole Grains and Cereals.** Have warm cereals such as oatmeal, grits, or Cream-of-Wheat. Avoid the packaged "quick" kinds which often are over-processed and have added sugars, salt and fat. Seven grain or multi-grain cereal is wonderful. This is seven whole grains that you cook like rice. Then you can eat it warm or cold. You can add it to your bread mix, mix it with ground beef, or use it in pasta salads. Seven grain cereal is worth a try. Also, look for Tabouli wheat salad in the rice section of your grocery store.

**Crackers.** Look for crackers that are made from whole grains, have low sodium and that are baked rather than fried. Bagel chips are also great, but make your own. Packaged bagel chips are often high in fat. Slice bagels thin, spray with cooking spray and add a sprinkle of parmesan cheese, or any seasonings. Bagel chips and salsa make a good combination.

*Potatoes.* Include sweet potatoes in your regular diet. Simply bake, slice and sprinkle with butter seasoning, nutmeg and salt. Or mash with skim milk and butter seasoning. Sweet potatoes are a terrific source of vitamins. Avoid sweet potato pie or patties which can be laden with butter, cream and nuts.

A good general rule to follow when choosing nutritious starches is to avoid *white* (that is, with the exception of starches that are naturally white such as potatoes.) White rice, bread and pasta are made from bleached, highly processed grains which are lower in vitamins, fiber and other nutrients. Go for rich, unbleached, minimally processed starches.

# WEEK 42: LOSE THE LARD

I n the second quarter, you did several things to reduce the fat in the meats that you eat. This week, we will take this concept one step further with these additional tips:

- Read back over the tips in Week 24, "Get the Lard Out." Improve on these where you can.

- Eat meat at only one meal a day, and have meatless days during the week.

- Limit your intake of beef and pork meals to twice a week. When you do eat meat, choose skinless, white meat chicken or fish.

- Avoid organ meats such as liver which are high in cholesterol.

- Much of the fat in a roast cooks off but ends up on your plate in the form of gravy. Here's the best way to make gravy: after the roast is done, pour hot water from boiled potatoes or vegetables into the roasting pan and scrape. Pour this liquid into a gravy separator and let sit in the refrigerator for a few moments. Pour the liquid into your sauce pan, leaving the grease in the gravy separator. Make a mixture of flour and water the consistency of pancake batter. Use about 1.5 tblsp flour to one cup of gravy liquid. Whisk the flour mixture into the gravy liquid, then heat, stirring, until it thickens.

- If you make broth from meats, separate it from the fat in the way described above. Or, save the water that you cook vegetable in for cooking rice, stir frys or soups.

- Grill, broil or bake most meats. Avoid pan frying which does not allow the fat to drain off. An excellent switch from fried chicken pieces is barbecued breast fillets. Most barbecue sauces are fat-free (although many are high in sugar.) Barbecue sauces can add a flavor punch without too many added calories.

- Cut your meat thinner. A quarter inch slice of turkey will look almost the same size as a half inch slice but will have half the fat and calories.

- Roast a turkey breast instead of a whole turkey. Don't stuff the turkey—the dressing will soak up too much fat. Cook the dressing in a separate baking dish and flavor with de-fatted broth.

- Consider meat more of a side dish, or even as a spice to a dish rather than the main course.

- Choose fresh fish or seafood to grill once or twice a week.

- Introduce beans into your diet. Legumes have suffered an undeserving bad reputation for unpleasant digestive effects. The trick to avoid this is to eat them regularly. If you eat beans twice a week, your stomach will develop the digestive enzymes necessary to break the beans down without producing gas. You should also soak overnight and discard the soaking liquid before cooking. Beans are great with rice, in soups and with pastas. When mashed, they also make a great base for a dip. There are dozens of varieties available, fresh, frozen, canned and dried. Dried beans or canned beans keep for months and should always be available in your pantry. Beans are a terrific protein source that is completely fat-free.

# WEEK 43: SMART SHOPPING

**G**rocery shopping can be your downfall or your ticket to success. This week you should concentrate on how to make your shopping trips help you reach your goal. Consider these for your next shopping trip:

- Go to the grocery store with your eating plan. Buy only what's on the plan.

- Most grocery stores are arranged so that the fresh, unprocessed foods are around the perimeter of the store. If this is the case in your store, stick with the perimeter and avoid the aisles.

- *Never* shop when hungry. Go right after dinner or another meal. This tip alone can make a huge difference in what you bring home from the grocery store.

- Shop for foods requiring preparation: chopping, peeling, cooking. Avoid foods (except fruit!) that you can eat right out of the bag.

- Every grocery store and market has a large non-fat foods area—the produce section! Start in the produce section and plan your meals around vegetables. Meat should be used as an accent for the meal, rather than the main course. Try a fruit, vegetable or spice that is new to you. Keep yourself open to new tastes.

- Shop often during the week and bring home fresh produce.

- Avoid preserved or processed foods. Try to stick with food in the most basic form. Processed food is more expensive, has added sugar, salt, fat and less nutrients. Fresh foods, however, do not have as long a shelf life. Frozen foods are a good alternative because they are frozen close to the time they are harvested and may be fresher than trucked produce.

- Skip the snack aisle completely. Don't even bother. Save yourself the expense, sodium, fat, calories and temptation.

- Try not to buy in large quantities. If you do, break it into serving size portions in baggies and store the extras in the freezer.

- Visit a local farmer's market rather than a supermarket. Local produce is usually fresher, tastier and less expensive.

- Allow yourself plenty of time to compare and read the Nutrition Facts labels.

- Be open minded and try something new. That is, of course, if it is a nutritious addition to your diet.

- On the other hand, vow not to try anything that you've never had before that is high in calories. It might turn out to be your next vice.

# WEEK 44: THE LEAN LIBRARY

T he average household in America has ten cookbooks. Chances are your cookbooks are outdated and not health centered. Explore new cookbooks that are based on the latest research in nutrition. Choose books featuring pastas, beans, vegetables, breads, spices and tofu.

Go through your favorite recipes that you have torn and saved from magazines or received from friends. Discard the ones that are very high in calories. You can attempt to modify some of the recipes using substitutions, but if they are a tremendous temptation, you may be better off discarding them. Be sure to do this after you've eaten a meal, when your resolve will be strong. Avoid the temptation to ask a friend for a recipe that you know is high in calories and/or fat.

Be a cookbook reader and be discriminating in what you choose. Try not to even open the ones that do not illustrate healthy recipes on the cover. Use the library. If there is a particular cookbook that is not in your library yet, ask the librarian. They can usually obtain it, either by purchase or by inter-library loans. Experiment and trade recipes with your support group.

Here are some excellent books that will help you slim down your cookbook library:

- *Live! Don't DIEt!* by Vicki Park. Dozens of great recipes, tips on cooking low-fat, and Vicki's inspiring story of losing 165 pounds.

- *Lean and Lovin' It!* by Don Mauer. Wonderfully inventive recipes by a man who has maintained a weight loss of 103 pounds.

- *Quick & Healthy Recipes and Ideas*, and *Quick & Healthy Volume II* by Brenda Ponichtera. Packed with information about nutrition and terrific, quick recipes. Both of these cookbooks should be in every kitchen.

You'll find more information on these and other cookbooks in the Bibliography in the Appendix.

One of the best sources of healthy cooking books is your local health food store. In addition to books, a great resource of healthy recipes and ideas is online computer forums. There are forums on healthy and vegetarian cooking where you can get hundreds of free recipes, and share your favorites with the group. You can also get computer CDs with literally thousands of recipes. On a CD, you can search for specific ingredients. For instance, say you have a bumper crop of summer squash, or it's on sale at the market. You can search on "squash" and find dozens of recipes.

Your county extension agent will also have many recipes, hints for leftovers and preserving and preparing foods. Spend this entire week revamping your outdated cooking library.

# WEEK 45: DAIRY DIET

Here is the second week devoted to decreasing your fat intake from dairy foods. Review Week 11: Dairy Don'ts and brush up on those tasks. Then, consider these:

- Gradually move away from mayonnaise. You can start by using mayonnaise that is 50% lower in fat. Try to substitute mayonnaise altogether with either mustard or plain yogurt. If you use mayonnaise in salad dressings, try using a mix of light mayonnaise and plain yogurt. If you introduce this gradually, you won't notice the difference. If you buy ranch style or creamy dressings, consider thinning the dressing a bit with skim milk.

- Rather than cheese or sour cream based dips, have salsa for dipping. Rather than chips with sour cream and onion dip, serve toasted pita chips with a spicy salsa.

- Modify your intake of butter. Powdered butter flavor or Butter Buds are great on steamed vegetables, baked potatoes or in sauces. Try jelly, applesauce, jam or honey on your toast instead. Margarine is just as high in calories and fat as butter is, however, it lacks the saturated fat of butter. You might find a "light" spread that is tasty. However, most light spreads are water based and do not melt or bake well (you'll end up with soggy toast or popcorn.) Keep your butter in the refrigerator, or better yet, in the freezer. If it's out on the counter and soft, it will be too tempting and easy to use.

- In cream sauces, substitute canned condensed milk for cream.

- Be cautious of coffee creamer. If you drink two cups of coffee a day, you may be getting as much as five grams of fat from the creamer. Try a low-fat, non-dairy creamer, non-fat condensed milk, or a low-fat flavored coffee as an alternative. Or, switch to an herbal tea.

- Rather than mixing cheese into a casserole, just sprinkle some on top. You will need to use much less. For a real cheese taste punch, use finely grated Romano, Asiago or Parmesan.

By reducing your fat intake from dairy products, you will also reduce your intake of saturated fats and cholesterol.

# WEEK 46: BODY BOOST

I t is time this week to increase your activity to at least 180 minutes per week. This should be divided roughly equally on most or all days of the week. This is the recommended minimum amount of exercise for the average American adult. By now you should have seen many benefits from regular activity. You probably FEEL muscles that you have not felt in years. You should feel the blood nourishing your fingers, shoulders, scalp, and skin.

Exercising is not something that you have to do. You don't have to lose weight either. But regular exercise will speed your progress, make you feel better, reduce stress, and increase your metabolism.

> *These are my new shoes. They're good shoes. They won't make you rich like me, they won't make you rebound like me, they definitely won't make you handsome like me. They'll only make you have shoes like me. That's it. -Charles Barkley, in a commercial for basketball shoes, 1993*

Take time this week to also review that other way of increasing your activity: those tiny things you can do all day long to burn calories. In general, you should be walking faster and more. You should not wait for the closest parking spaces. You should always take the stairs up three flights rather than using the elevator. Try to get up from your chair every hour and do three minutes of brisk walking. In an eight hour workday, that's 24 minutes of activity that qualifies as exercise. All these things, when done consistently every day, add up. Here are few more examples:

- Be a scout leader.
- Adopt a Mile on a street and keep it clean. Enlist the help of a child or neighbor.
- Join a local sport team such as bowling, tennis, baseball. Or, organize a local team with neighbors and friends.
- Go ice skating.
- Ride a bike to the store.
- Go horseback riding.
- Play a game of pickup basketball with the kids.

Remember that exercise not only burns calories, but regular exercise increases your resting metabolic rate. Muscle tissue burns more calories than fat. Your body and muscles are meant to be used. Exercise will bring oxygen and nutrients to every part of your body while moving waste materials out. Your skin and hair will look better, you will move more gracefully, you will be more alert, and you will feel good about yourself.

# WEEK 47: I GOTTA NEW ATTITUDE

W e are actually living in an environment that is unnatural to our appetites and metabolism. Your body was not meant to resist food. When food was truly scarce, those with the biggest appetites were the fittest, and those with the slowest metabolisms survived famines. Our country has been blessed (or plagued) with an abundance of food. Our great, great grandfathers could not have imagined that overeating would be such a significant problem. Today, in three minutes for three dollars you can get 3,000 calories from a fast food window. A century ago, a 3,000 calorie meal would have taken a full day (or more) of hunting, gathering and preparation by the entire family. You would have to *work* and *use calories* to eat. Today, you can get a 3,000 calorie meal (and that is 30% more than the average adult should eat in a day) for less than one hour's work at minimum wage and with little or no burning of calories.

Even our pets have diet foods and are overweight. We should be thankful that we are not starving. In our society, we must practice refusal of food to stay healthy. This is something our bodies were not conditioned to do, mentally or physically.

We need to adjust our view of food relative to the everyday marketing efforts of a multi-billion dollar food industry. "You deserve a break today" is a message that tells you it's not only OK, it's a reward to eat a high-fat meal. This is not what you deserve— you deserve health, energy and the self-esteem that comes with controlling your weight. This is not to say that you will never be able to eat another cheeseburger again. On the contrary, you need to eat the foods that you love, but, you need to control the portions and number of times that you indulge. You can also make smart substitutions and still be satisfied.

*So live that you wouldn't be ashamed to sell the family parrot to the town gossip.*
*– Will Rogers*

You can have your Big Mac, but with a salad and water instead of fries and a cola. Yes, you do deserve a break today: a break from overeating, a break from high-fat, high-calorie foods and a break from that vicious cycle of overeating and guilt.

Rather than focus our time and energy on obtaining food, as we had to hundreds of years ago, we must now change our focus. We don't have to spend ten hours a day hunting, gathering, growing, preparing and preserving food. We now have more time to nurture our families, to learn, to improve our standard of living, and to concentrate on our spirituality. We have the weapon of knowledge to help us modify our eating habits to live healthy lives in today's society. By being informed on nutrition and closely aware of your body's needs, you can adjust your food quality and quantity. You *can* live healthier and happier without feeling deprived or starved. You *can* control your life so that your primary focus is living, not food.

Spend this week concentrating on changing your focus and attitude. You are not on a diet. You are no longer living the lifestyle of an overweight person. You are in control and will be for the rest of your life.

# WEEK 48: CRUSH THE CRAVE

L ast quarter, we looked at problem areas and you should have pinpointed one particular food that triggers overeating. You started on a plan to get that problem under control. Use this week to tighten up your control over that trigger. If you feel you are already in control of the problem, use this week to identify and tackle another.

We have looked at the circumstances that might bring on uncontrolled eating of a problem food. This week you will devise a specific plan to gain even more control. Throughout the year, we have used similar guidelines to gain moderation. Eliminate the problem food

*I couldn't help it. I can resist everything except temptation.*
*- Oscar Wilde, from Lady Windermere's Fan*

gradually. Or, rather than eliminate it, get your portions sizes and occurrences under control. You are in control now, and you have the power to methodically chip away at this problem. Make a plan, record it in your food journal and keep your promise to yourself. Here's a sample plan of attack:

- Problem food: ice cream, currently eat two cups five times per week.

- This week: have 2 cups of a non-fat frozen yogurt twice, and 2 cups of ice cream three times.

- Three weeks from now: Reduce serving size from two cups to one.

- Six weeks from now: Reduce number of times per week. Frozen yogurt two times, ice cream once.

- Nine weeks from now: Frozen yogurt once a week and ice cream once.

- Twelve weeks from now: Reduce serving size to one half cup.

You can make this in even smaller steps over a longer period of time. If you find that it is extremely difficult, spread it out. Your goal is to get this under control and it is better if you do it successfully taking two years than if you fail many times in one year.

To help you through those cravings, pick up your list of Fun Things, or your To-Do list. Try one of these diversions:

- Chew a piece of gum.

- Ask yourself, am I really hungry or am I frustrated, bored, depressed or angry? Take care of the cause, don't make it worse.

- Call your support partner.

- Take the stairs for two flights up and down and then reconsider.

- Try on your old "fat" clothes

- Go shopping for a bathing suit.

- Run an errand.

- Put on your headphones and play your favorite CD or listen to a book on tape.

- Ask yourself and write down how will you feel if you give in, and how will you feel if you maintain control.

- Brush your teeth.

You should gradually reduce your intake of this problem food so that by the end of the year it no longer controls you. You will be able to eat a reasonable portion of it as a treat on occasion. But, if at the end of year you have followed the *Live It!* plan, your cravings for these high-calorie and high-fat foods will be substantially lowered.

# WEEK 49: THE EVENING HOURS

Y ou've come a long way. You should have control of 12 hours of your 16 waking hours. If not, look back at the weeks devoted to taking control of meals and snacking. Review those weeks, and renew your commitment.

The evening is a wonderfully relaxing time of day. Time for family, reflection on the day and planning for tomorrow. Unfortunately it is also a time when many folks sit in front of the TV eating and drinking. If this is a particularly bad time of the day for you, you may want

> *It's all right letting yourself go, as long as you can let yourself back. -Mick Jagger*

to change not only your eating habits, but also what you normally do after dinner. There are many great things to do during these hours. Here is a mix of alternatives to snacking and watching television:

- Brush your teeth right after dinner. This will cleanse your mouth and reduce your urge to snack.

- Have a cup of tea. A hot beverage can be soothing and filling.

- Take a walk.

- Read a book.

- Go to bed earlier. Almost everyone can use more sleep.

- Take a hot bath an hour before bedtime.

- Stargaze.

- Have sex.

- Plan your activities and food for tomorrow in your food journal.

- Make lunch and snacks for the next day for yourself and the family.

- Call that friend or family member that you haven't spoken to in a long while, while long distance rates are low.


Remember your tools when you are tempted to overeat: your goals, your food journal, your To-Do list and your List of Fun Things. Put them to work for you.

# WEEK 50: DO YOU DO TOFU?

T his week we'll look at reducing our dependance on meat. Most Americans have grown up with each meal centered around a meat entree. This is more a habit than a dietary necessity. The most important dietary challenge Americans face is to cut down on the excess fats in our diet, particularly saturated fats which come from animal products. Meat should be viewed as a compliment to the occasional meal, and not the main course at every meal. When choosing alternatives to meat, be careful that you do not replace your meat portions with too much cheese. Cheese can be dangerously high in saturated fats and calories. You do not want to trade one bad habit for another.

An excellent protein substitute for meat is tofu. Tofu can be cooked in any way imaginable—from stir fry to shishkabobs. It can be blended to form a base for dips and dressings. By now you should have an open mind to new healthier alternatives. There are several excellent cookbooks featuring tofu, and more restaurants are offering tofu dishes. Be sure to try it in several different ways before passing judgment. One of the best qualities of tofu is that it is so versatile. The taste and texture of tofu can be dramatically different from one dish to the next.

Here are some other meatless entree ideas:

- A pizza topped with mushrooms and black olives. Use shredded mozzarella made from part-skim milk.

- A filling potato soup.

- A stir fry with Portabella mushrooms, spring onions, Shanghai bok choy, and water chestnuts on jasmine rice.

- Rice and beans, such as black beans and rice, or Cajun red beans and rice. Beans are an excellent source of protein. They are easy to have on hand, either dried or canned.

- A great chef salad with greens, tomatoes, peppers, mushrooms, a sprinkle of parmesan cheese and a ranch dressing made with low-fat mayonnaise.

- Lasagna made with mushrooms or spinach.

- Any pasta with a tomato-based sauce.

- A garden burger. These are made from food such as rice, soy beans, other legumes, TVP, mushrooms, whole grains with other vegetables and spices. Many restaurants are now serving their own special version of a garden burger. You can also get them in the frozen section of the grocery store. Try a couple different brands to find one you like.

If you are not used to vegetarian cooking, seek out a few references on vegetarian cuisine. Here are two of my favorites:

- *Lean Bean Cuisine,* by Jay Solomon, is an excellent cookbook and bean reference guide.

- *How to Feed a Vegetarian,* by Suzanne D'Avalon is a wonderful book for those who are new to vegetarian cooking.

You'll find more information on these and other references in the Bibliography Appendix.

# WEEK 51: WHERE DO YOU GO FROM HERE?

T he beauty of the *Live It!* Plan is that you do not have to move into that dangerous phase of "dieting" called "maintenance." This is often the time when dieters fail. They lose weight while on a restrictive diet, then either lose control or do not have the tools that they need to eat healthy for the rest of their lives. But because you have not been on a "diet" and you have adjusted to a healthy lifestyle, there is no need to make an adjustment for maintenance.

Do you need to continue to use a food journal? Do you need to continue to track your weight and watch those calories and plan every meal? Each individual will have a different answer to this question. You may be able to use the habits and tools you have developed this year without the need of a daily food journal. You may have developed a mental mindset of planning and estimating and controlling what you eat. On the other hand, you may need a daily reminder to keep focused on healthy living. Rather than daily planning and recording, you may want to simply set aside an hour each week to review a week in your food journal.

By all means, review your *Live It!* book periodically. Use it to refresh your skills. Monitor your weight, either by the scale or by the fit of your clothes. Be careful about seasonal clothing however. Your winter clothes that you just bought may be smaller than the summer clothes you wore nine months ago. You may slowly gain weight over the summer and then surprisingly not be able to zip your winter pants. Keep one pair of jeans or pants that you can wear on one day each week, year round. When these become snug, take action. It is much easier to tackle two pounds than to face twenty.

An excellent way to stay reminded of your past poor lifestyle is to stay in touch with your support group. You can provide invaluable hope and motivation to those who are where you were one year ago. As you are helping someone else achieve success, you will reinforce your commitment to yourself. As each year goes by, you can be living proof that control is possible.

# WEEK 52: THE YEAR IN REVIEW

Y ou've made it! If you focused each week on the task at
hand, then you are living a healthier life with a manageable
weight. You've mastered the art of moderation and control.
You should not only be thinner, but more alert, more energetic and
healthier. This week is a review of the entire year. Have you met
your goal? If you've followed most of the guidelines and used
many of the tips, you should have. Perhaps you met your goal, but
still have more weight to lose. If so, simply spend another year
with the food journal, fine tuning each week and slowly adjusting
to your final weight. You may want to choose only those weeks
that need refinement.

Let's review last quarter:

**Dinner:** Keep some vegetable stock on hand to add to rices,
or as a base for a soup. When you trim your vegetables, put the
stems and leaves that are not eaten into a pan and simmer. Remove
the solids, and store the broth in the refrigerator.

Don't Diet—*Live It!*

***Bring on the Bread:*** Try an herb bread rather than cheese or sweet bread.

***Loose the Lard:*** Try a couple of different gourmet, spicy mustards in place of mayonnaise.

***Smart Shopping:*** Keep your shopping list on a page in your food journal. You should always have it with you, and keeping it in your food journal will encourage you to keep a healthy grocery list.

***The Lean Library:*** Share a favorite recipe or lean cookbook with your support partner.

***Dairy Diet:*** Instead of ice cream, have sherbet, ice milk or frozen yogurt.

***Body Boost:*** Attend a local high school basketball, baseball, football or soccer game.

***I Gotta New Attitude:*** For the next 24 hours, pretend that everything you do is videotaped, and that someone you respect is going to view the tape.

***Crush the Crave:*** If you *really* want it, and *are hungry*, then go ahead and eat it—in moderation. Don't beat yourself up. Enjoy it and enjoy the fact that you *can* eat your favorite foods in moderation.

***The Evening Hours:*** The perfect time for a bit of net surfing. Look at Appendix D: Internet Sites of Interest.

***Better Proteins:*** Try Texturized Vegetable Protein (TVP) in any casserole in place of ground meat. You can get this at a health food store.

***Where Do You Go From Here?:*** Stay in touch with your support group. They need you, and you need them.

No doubt during the year some days were better than others. That's life. With the tools and new habits that you now have, you can adjust to those challenges. You cannot control everything around you, but you can control, to a great extent, your weight, health and longevity. And with these things come contentment and the ability for happiness for yourself and your family.

This is a week for congratulations, savoring life, reflecting on the success of the year, and reinforcing the goals that brought you here. If you are reading this, but are still in the early weeks of the plan, visualize the success of this final week now. It can be yours.

I sincerely hope that the *Live It!* Plan has helped you gain the control that you have been seeking all your life. I'd like to hear about your success, and any special tips that you've used to achieve that success. Please write c/o White Papers Press, P.O. Box 72294, Marietta, GA 30007, or send an email to wpp@mindspring.com.

# REFERENCE

# SECTION

# APPENDIX A: THE FOOD GUIDE PYRAMID

The Food Guide Pyramid is a valuable result of years of nutritional research on the American diet. It was derived from many controlled studies and offers the best information on how to eat to stay healthy. The following table illustrates the Food Guide Pyramid. Note that the lower number of servings per day is for a smaller individual and the higher number in the range of servings per day is for the taller, larger framed person.

# Food Guide Pyramid

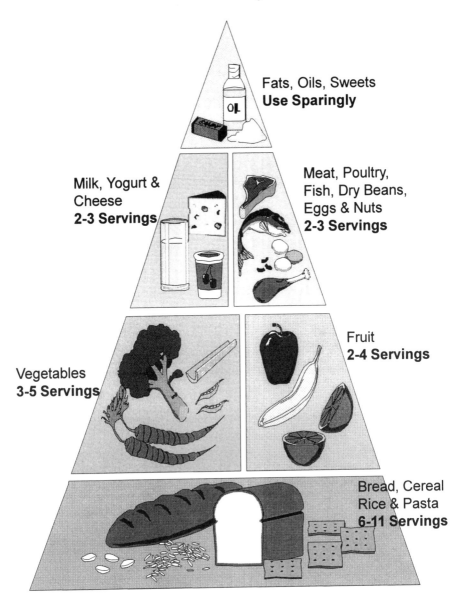

Fats, Oils, Sweets
**Use Sparingly**

Milk, Yogurt & Cheese
**2-3 Servings**

Meat, Poultry, Fish, Dry Beans, Eggs & Nuts
**2-3 Servings**

Vegetables
**3-5 Servings**

Fruit
**2-4 Servings**

Bread, Cereal Rice & Pasta
**6-11 Servings**

Source: Using the Food Guide Pyramid: A Resource for Nutrition Educators U.S. Department of Agriculture Food, Nutrition and Consumer Services Center for Nutrition Policy and Promotion, 1995

# APPENDIX B: SIMPLE SUBSTITUTIONS

Most of these substitutions are culled from the preceding chapters. They are assembled here in a checklist format. Try each one, and check them off as you go. Making some painless substitutions in your daily diet can add up to astounding results. Just one 12 ounce cola has 155 calories. *One per day for a year equals 16 pounds.* You don't have to eat all imitation fat-free, low-calorie substitutes. Eat real food, but try some of these substitutions to increase you chances of success.

Do not underestimate the power of these little changes. Take some time to review the ones that we've already seen. Seriously consider each one and try to make it fit into your life. Some are deceptively simple, but can have tremendous results. For instance, switching from mayonnaise to mustard on two sandwiches a week can save 10,400 calories and 1,144 grams of fat this year. That alone is three pounds. This is how to chip away those pounds ounce by ounce. That's exactly how they got on you, and that's exactly how they'll melt away.

|   | Rather than: | Try this (equal or smaller portion): |
|---|---|---|
| ❑ | adult menu | child's menu, or the appetizer menu |
| ❑ | apple pie | apple crisp with no pie crust |
| ❑ | bacon | Canadian bacon |

| | Rather than: | Try this (equal or smaller portion): |
|---|---|---|
| ❑ | beef, ground | ground beef cooked well, drained, and squeezed in paper towels. Add an extender such as oatmeal, texturized vegetable protein or crushed crackers. |
| ❑ | beer, regular | light beer |
| ❑ | bread, cheese | herb bread |
| ❑ | bread, white | wheat or whole grain bread |
| ❑ | broth, chicken or beef | fat-free canned broths, or vegetable broths to flavor stir frys, soups and rices |
| ❑ | butter on toast | apple butter or preserves |
| ❑ | cake with frosting | angel food cake with fresh fruit sprinkled with powdered sugar |
| ❑ | canned tuna in oil | canned albacore tuna in water |
| ❑ | cheese, cheddar on salads | finely grated Romano or Parmesan cheese, or low-fat cheddar cheese |
| ❑ | cheese, cream | Neufchatel cheese or cream cheese with one-third fewer calories |
| ❑ | cheese, ricotta | low-fat cottage cheese |
| ❑ | cheese, sliced on a sandwich | low-fat or fat-free sliced cheese |
| ❑ | chicken, fried | boneless, skinless chicken breast grilled and basted with barbecue sauce |

| | Rather than: | Try this (equal or smaller portion): |
|---|---|---|
| ❏ | chocolate candy | lollipop or butterscotch, low-fat chocolate milk, fat-free, chocolate pudding made with skim milk |
| ❏ | chocolate syrup | powdered chocolate milk mix |
| ❏ | coffee cream or Half & Half | non-fat dairy creamer |
| ❏ | cookies, macaroon or chocolate chip | vanilla wafers, graham crackers, animal cookies, fat-free fruit newtons, or ginger snaps |
| ❏ | corn chips or potato chips | toasted pita triangles or toasted bagel chips |
| ❏ | cream in sauces | evaporated skim milk |
| ❏ | croissant | plain bagel or English muffin |
| ❏ | dessert, creamy | sugar-free pudding made with 1% milk |
| ❏ | dessert, sweet | fat-free candies or Jell-O |
| ❏ | dip, ranch or sour cream based | salsa |
| ❏ | dressing cooked inside the turkey | dressing cooked in a separate baking dish so that it won't soak up the fat inside the turkey. Flavor with defatted broth. |
| ❏ | egg, whole | egg whites only, or two whites to one yolk |

| | Rather than: | Try this (equal or smaller portion): |
|---|---|---|
| ❑ | fried | broiled, grilled, poached or baked |
| ❑ | fruit, canned in syrup | fresh fruit |
| ❑ | granola cereal | Grape Nuts cereal |
| ❑ | hamburger, quarter pound | junior burger or veggie burger |
| ❑ | ice cream | fat-free frozen yogurt, sherbet, a popsicle, or berries topped with Cool Whip |
| ❑ | ice cream cone, large waffle | small sugar cone |
| ❑ | large order (of any item) | small order |
| ❑ | lunch, fast food | yogurt or low-fat cottage cheese for lunch one day a week |
| ❑ | mayonnaise | light mayonnaise or mustard for a sandwich; plain yogurt for dressings or dips, or a mixture of mayonnaise and plain yogurt |
| ❑ | meat, in stir fry | Portabella mushrooms, and a tablespoon of oyster sauce |
| ❑ | meat, pork or beef | skinless chicken breasts, turkey breast or fish |
| ❑ | milk, whole | skim or 1% |

| | Rather than: | Try this (equal or smaller portion): |
|---|---|---|
| ❑ | nuts on ice cream or yogurt | Grape Nuts cereal |
| ❑ | nuts, chocolate chips or sugar in recipes | Half the amount, or try carob chips in place of chocolate. |
| ❑ | oil in baked goods | applesauce |
| ❑ | pasta salad | add an equal amount of vegetables such as blanched spinach, broccoli, celery, peppers, asparagus, artichoke hearts or snow peas: Shake dressing on top just before eating, otherwise it will soak into pasta and you will need more to taste. |
| ❑ | pepperoni | Canadian bacon |
| ❑ | popcorn, with butter | air-popped popcorn with powdered butter flavor |
| ❑ | popsicle | freeze orange juice in plastic popsicle containers |
| ❑ | potato chips | pretzels, baked potato chips |
| ❑ | potato, baked with sour cream and butter | baked potato with salsa, sun dried tomatoes, or seasoned salt |
| ❑ | potato, baked with sour cream and butter | mashed potatoes mashed with skim milk and one teaspoon of butter per potato. Sprinkle on Butter Buds. |

Don't Diet—*Live It!*

| | Rather than: | Try this (equal or smaller portion): |
|---|---|---|
| ❑ | potatoes, french fried | baked "fries": Thinly slice an unpeeled raw potato. Coat with two egg whites mixed with one tablespoon of seasoned salt. Place on a single layer on a sprayed cookie sheet. Cook for 40 minutes at 400 degrees, turning occasionally. |
| ❑ | sandwich, submarine with pastrami, may-onnaise, cheese | submarine with sliced turkey, tomato, lettuce, onion and mustard |
| ❑ | sauce, cream based | tomato based sauce |
| ❑ | sauce, tartar | cocktail sauce |
| ❑ | sausage biscuit | Canadian bacon and English muffin |
| ❑ | sour cream | unflavored yogurt |
| ❑ | steak, one inch thick | half inch thick steak |
| ❑ | syrup | dip your waffle or pancake in applesauce with a small amount of maple syrup, or sprinkle powdered sugar or cinnamon sugar |

# APPENDIX C: BIBLIOGRAPHY

Barnard, Neal D: *Eat Right, Live Longer: Using the Natural Power of Foods to Age-Proof Your Body*, Crown Pub, January 1997, ISBN: 0517887789

Barthalomew, Mel: *Square Foot Gardening*, Rodale Press, 1994, ISBN: 9994957996

Blonz, Edward R.: *The Really Simple, No Nonsense Nutrition Guide*, Conari Press, ISBN 0-943233-45-3.

Center for Science in the Public Interest: *Nutrition Action Health Letter*

Chopra, Deepak: *Perfect Weight: The Complete Mind/Body Program for Achieving and Maintaining Your Ideal Weight*, Harmony Books, October, 1994, ISBN: 0517599228

D'Avalon, Suzanne, *How to Feed a Vegetarian: Help for Non-Vegetarian Cooks*, Placidly Amid the Noise, 1996, 0965094103

Ferguson, James M.: *Habits Not Diets: The Secret to Lifetime Weight Control*, Bull Pub Co, May, 1989, ISBN: 0915950855

Gullo, Stephen P.: *Thin Tastes Better: Control Your Food Triggers and Lose Weight Without Feeling Deprived*, Dell Pub Co, March, 1996, ISBN: 0440222311

Fletcher, Anne M.: *Thin for Life: 10 Keys to Success from People Who Have Lost Weight and Kept It Off*, Chapters Pub Ltd, February, 1995, ISBN: 1881527603

Johnson, Heidi: *Deliciously Simple: The Smart Way to Cook*, 1995, - (888)226-9392.

Jordan, Peg: *How the New Food Labels Can Save Your Life*, Michael Wiese Productions, 1994.

Kraus, Barbara: *Calories and Carbohydrates*, 11Th/Rev Edition, Signet, May, 1995, ISBN: 0451183355

Mauer, Don: *Lean and Lovin' It!: Exceptionally Delicious Recipes for Low-Fat Living and Permanent Weight Loss*, Chapters, 1996, ISBN: 1881527972.

Park, Vicki, *Live! Don't DIEt: The Low-fat Cookbook That Can Change Your Life*, Warner, 1995, ISBN 0-4466729-7.

Papazian, Ruth: *Healthful Snacks for the Chip-and-Dip Crowd*, FDA Web site, http://www.fda.gov/

Ponichtera, Brenda J., R.D.: *Quick & Healthy Recipes and Ideas: For people who say they don't have time to cook healthy meals*, Scaledown Publishing, Inc, 1994, ISBN: 0962916005.

Ponichtera, Brenda J., R.D.: *Quick & Healthy Volume II*, Scaledown Publishing, Inc, 1995, ISBN: 0962916013.

Saltos, Etta: *The Food Pyramid-Food Label Connection*, FDA Consumer, June 1993.

Spiller, Dr. Gene and Madison, Deborah: *The Superpyramid Eating Program: Introducing the Revolutionary Five New Food Groups*, Times Books, January 1993, ISBN: 0812920562

Solomon, Jay: *Lean Bean Cuisine: Over 100 Tasty Meatless Recipes from Around the World*, Prima Pub, July, 1994, ISBN: 1559584386

Somer, Elizabeth: *Food & Mood: The Complete Guide to Eating Well and Feeling Your Best*, Henry Holt, April 1996, ISBN: 0805045627

U.S. Department of Agriculture and U.S. Department of Health and Human Services: *Dietary Guidelines for Americans*, Fourth Edition, 1995.

U.S. Department of Agriculture, Food Nutrition, and Consumer Services, Center for Nutrition Policy and Promotion: *Using the Food Guide Pyramid: A Resource for Nutrition Educators.*

U. S. Food and Drug Administration: *FDA's New Food Label.*

U. S. Food and Drug Administration:*The Facts about Weight Loss Products and Programs,* FDA/FTC/NAAG Brochure, 1992.

Vartabedian, Roy E and Matthews, Kathy: *Nutripoints: The Breakthrough Point System for Optimal Nutrition,* Harper, February 1991, ISBN: 0061099171

# APPENDIX D: INTERNET SITES OF INTEREST

Internet sites come and go. At the time of printing, these were well-established sites dedicated to health and/or weight management.

**http://www1.mhv.net/~donn/diet.html**
A funky address, but well worth finding! Articles and links to diet tips, low-fat recipes, news, support, FAQs, exercise, healthy eating, new weight loss products, nutrition, and much more. Start here or at the site below.

**http://www.blonz.com/blonz/index.html**
The site includes information on nutrition, food science, foods, fitness and health. An excellent site to start your surfing. Includes links to many of the sites listed below.

**http://www.healthyideas.com**
Prevention Magazine's website. Create your own weight loss program, find healthy recipes, a forum and information on exercise.

**http://www.nutribase.com**
The NutriBase Web Site features an interactive on-line database of 19,344 food items that you can view, rank, query and search by food names. This database includes 3,160 menu items from 71 restaurants. Also features a weight-loss calculator, a calorie requirements calculator, "desirable" weight and body fat content charts, a directory of 1,376 food and supplement makers, a listing

of healthy food substitutions, a glossary of foods and cooking terms, toll-free numbers for food makers, and 1,000 quotes and tips for dieters.

## http://www.cspinet.org

Home page for the Center for Science in the Public Interest (CSPI), a nonprofit education and advocacy organization that focuses on improving the safety and nutritional quality of our food supply and on reducing the carnage caused by alcoholic beverages. Very informative.

## http://www.richardsimmons.com/

Dedicated to the cause? I think so. You just have to visit Richard's site.

## http://www.shapeup.org/sua/

Provides latest information about safe weight management and physical fitness by Dr. C. Everett Koop.

## http://www.tops.org/main/guide/brochure.html

Provides members with information, motivation and fellowship in attaining and maintaining their physician-prescribed weight goals.

## http://www.caloriecontrol.org/

Representing the low-calorie and reduced-fat food and beverage industry; site includes the calorie counter calculator.

## http://www.cyberdiet.com/

Answers questions about adopting a healthy lifestyle which includes a do-it-yourself nutritional profile to let you calculate your ideal body weight.

http://www.diettalk.com/
Provides chat room, bulletin board, and recipe area for people struggling with the everyday issues of dieting.

http://dmi-www.mc.duke.edu/dfc/home.html
The Duke University Diet & Fitness Center.

http://www.nal.usda.gov/
U.S. Department of Agriculture.

http://www.fda.gov/
Food and Drug Administration Home Page.

http://www.nsf.org/
Homepage for the National Sanitation Foundation, a non-profit organization active in insuring the safety and purity of foods and water.

http://www.pueblo.gsa.gov/
Consumer Information Center. Text versions of hundreds of the best free federal consumer publications available.

http://www.nal.usda.gov/fnic/foodcomp/
Look Up values in the USDA Nutrient Database for Standard Reference.

# APPENDIX E: THE YEAR AT A GLANCE

| | First Quarter | | Second Quarter | | Third Quarter | | Fourth Quarter |
|---|---|---|---|---|---|---|---|
| 1 | Put It in Writing | 14 | Make It Last | 27 | Let's Do Lunch | 40 | Dinner |
| 2 | Breakfast of Champions | 15 | Dare You Dine Out? | 28 | Good Things Are Green | 41 | Bring on the Bread |
| 3 | What's Your Dream? | 16 | Produce the Produce | 29 | The Healthy Kitchen | 42 | Loose the Lard |
| 4 | Planning | 17 | What's Your Pleasure? | 30 | Unfinished Business | 43 | Smart Shopping |
| 5 | The Mid-Morning Hours | 18 | Beverage Leverage | 31 | Growing Groceries | 44 | The Lean Library |
| 6 | The Buddy System | 19 | Too Much of a Good Thing | 32 | Tame Your Sweet Tooth | 45 | Dairy Diet |
| 7 | Get the Skinny | 20 | Wanna Dance? | 33 | Move It and Lose It | 46 | Body Boost |
| 8 | The Water Way | 21 | Get Out of That Rut | 34 | Celebrate! | 47 | I Gotta New Attitude |
| 9 | Get the Lead Out | 22 | Lotsa Pasta | 35 | Shave the Crave | 48 | Crush the Crave |
| 10 | Rate Your Weight | 23 | Watch Those Dollars Roll In | 36 | Afternoon Snacking | 49 | The Evening Hours |
| 11 | Dairy Don'ts | 24 | Get the Lard Out | 37 | Loosen Up and Chill Out | 50 | Do You Do Tofu? |
| 12 | Set the Stage for Success | 25 | Go Low Sodium | 38 | Go Fish | 51 | Where Do You Go From Here? |
| 13 | First Quarter Review | 26 | Second Qtr Review | 39 | Third Quarter Review | 52 | The Year in Review |

# INDEX